CW01476017

Shooting at Sandy нооk Elementary School

The Adam Lanza Report

November 2014

Connecticut Office of the Child Advocate

Published by OccupyBawlStreet.com Press

ISBN-13: 978-0692339022

ISBN-10: 0692339027

Subject Headings:

1. Law Enforcement
2. School Violence
3. Mental Illness
4. Child Welfare
5. Child Advocacy
6. Child Protective Services
7. Adam Lanza

Copyright Notice

Cover, Title & Copyright Page © 2014 OccupyBawlStreet.com Press

The document following this notice is a work of the State of Connecticut in the public domain and is not subject to copyright protection in the United States. Foreign copyrights may apply.

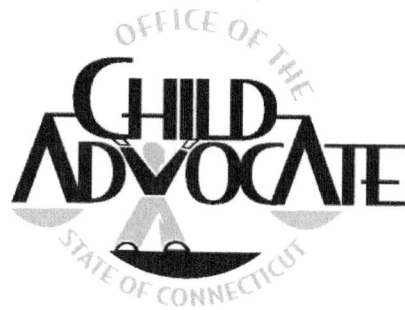

SHOOTING AT SANDY HOOK ELEMENTARY SCHOOL

REPORT OF THE OFFICE OF THE CHILD ADVOCATE

November 21, 2014

DEDICATION

The authors of this report submit this work with acknowledgement of the 27 individuals murdered on December 14, 2012, and the terrible and incalculable loss suffered by all victims. Authors convey condolences for these losses and the grief that continues to be felt by the victims, families, and the community. We acknowledge and honor the lives of the twenty first graders who died at Sandy Hook Elementary School; they have been the sole reason for this report.

Avielle

Ana

Allison

Benjamin

Caroline

Catherine

Charlotte

Chase

Daniel

Dylan

Emilie

Grace

Jack

Jesse

Josephine

Jessica

James

Madeleine

Noah

Olivia

STATEMENT FROM THE AUTHORS

In January, 2013, the Office of the Child Advocate was directed by the Connecticut Child Fatality Review Panel to prepare a report that would focus on Adam Lanza (hereinafter referred to as AL), and include a review of the circumstances that pre-dated his commission of mass murder at Sandy Hook Elementary School. The charge was to develop any recommendations for public health system improvement that emanated from the review. Authors of this report focused on AL's developmental, educational, and mental health profile over time, the services he received from various community providers, and ultimately his condition prior to his actions on December 14, 2012.

Authors looked for any warning signs, red flags, or other lessons that could be learned from a review of AL's life. It was not the primary purpose of this investigation to explicitly examine the role of guns in the Sandy Hook shootings. However, the conclusion cannot be avoided that access to guns is relevant to an examination of ways to improve the public health. Access to assault weapons with high capacity magazines did play a major role in this and other mass shootings in recent history. Our emphasis on AL's developmental trajectory and issues of mental illness should not be understood to mean that these issues were considered more important than access to these weapons or that we do not consider such access to be a critical public health issue.

It is important to state at the outset that this report is crafted with recognition of the lives lost on December 14, and authors have a deep sense of compassion for the families of the children and adults who were murdered by AL. To honor the terrible loss of life, authors strove to create a comprehensive and candid report that we hope will inform approaches to making other children, families, and communities safer in the future.

This report will identify missed opportunities in the life of AL. Authors underscore however that only AL was responsible for his murderous actions at Sandy Hook. ***There can be no direct line drawn between one entity or person's actions and a mass murder.*** This report cannot and does not answer the question of "why" AL committed murder. This report focuses on how to identify and assess youth from a very young age, the importance of effective mental health and educational service delivery, and the necessity of cross-system communication amongst professionals charged with the care of children.

Additionally, because the work of this report tracks AL from birth to the mass shooting the authors described AL in what appear to be human terms. Authors acknowledge that the telling of AL's story may be painful for some readers, especially those irrevocably harmed by his terrible actions. However, the report required a review of AL's life to address interventions and services that could have and should have been delivered over the course of his life. This report does not seek to draw any link between mental illness and violence, or between persons with autism and violence. As stated later in the report, there are millions of individuals with mental illness or developmental challenges in this country and worldwide, and a very small percentage of these individuals will engage in any act of violence, much less violence on a horrific scale. AL was an individual with mental illness and he was an individual who was diagnosed as having Autism Spectrum Disorder. This report outlines *this* story and makes recommendations accordingly. It is vital to note that AL was completely *untreated* in the years before the shooting and did not receive sustained, effective services during critical periods of his life, and it is this story that the report seeks to tell. .

Table of Contents

ACKNOWLEDGEMENTS

Many individuals contributed to the development of this report.

Primary Authors Include

Sarah Healy Eagan, J.D., Child Advocate State of Connecticut, Office of the Child Advocate
Faith VosWinkel, M.S.W., Assistant Child Advocate, Office of the Child Advocate
Julian D. Ford, Ph.D, Dept. of Psychiatry, Center for Trauma Recovery and Juvenile Justice University of Connecticut Health Center
Christopher Lyddy, L.C.S.W., C.O.O., Advanced Trauma Solutions, Inc.
Harold I. Schwartz, M.D., Psychiatrist-in-chief, Institute of Living, Hartford Hospital, Connecticut
Andrea Spencer, Ph.D., Dean, School of Education, Pace University

Additional Contributors Include

Kirsten Bechtel, M.D., Yale New Haven Hospital
Kathleen Costello, MSW Candidate, University of Connecticut School of Social Work
Jeffrey Goldberg, Copy Editor
James W. Loomis, Ph.D., The Center for Children with Special Needs, Glastonbury, CT
Felicia McGinniss, Law Student, University of Connecticut School of Law
Michael D. Powers, Psy.D., Director, CCSN: The Center for Children with Special Needs & The Center for Independence, Glastonbury, CT
Colleen Shaddox, Communications consultant
Paul Weigle, M.D., Child and Adolescent Psychiatrist, Natchaug Hospital

Additional Acknowledgements

The Office of the Child Advocate would also like to extend thanks to the following individuals and organizations for assisting with the development of this report:
Connecticut State Police
Federal Bureau of Investigation
Members of the State Child Fatality Review Panel
Nina Rovinelli Heller, Ph.D., Professor, University of Connecticut School of Social Work
Patricia Llodra, First Selectwoman, Town of Newtown
State's Attorney's Office, Judicial District of Danbury
U.S. Attorney's Office, District of Connecticut

EXECUTIVE SUMMARY

On Friday, December 14, 2012, our state and nation were stunned by the overwhelming tragedy at Sandy Hook Elementary School where twenty children and six educators were shot in their school. AL, who had already shot his mother in their home, also shot himself.

In the immediate aftermath of this terrible event, state and federal law enforcement agencies began investigating the circumstances leading up to the shooting. On January 30, 2013, the State Child Fatality Review Panel (CFRP)--charged with reviewing the sudden and unexpected death of children-directed the state Office of the Child Advocate (OCA) to investigate the circumstances leading to the death of the children at Sandy Hook, with a focus on any public health recommendations that may emanate from a review of the shooter's personal history. The Office of the Child Advocate, with the assistance of co-authors and consultants, reviewed numerous subjects pertinent to the charge from the CFRP, including:

- The mental health, developmental and social history of AL from his birth to the days before the shootings at Sandy Hook Elementary School.
- The educational record of AL, including documentation of needs and services provided.
- The medical history of AL from childhood to adulthood.
- Relevant laws regarding special education and confidentiality of records and how these laws implicate professional obligations and practices.

OCA began a comprehensive collection and review of records related to the life of AL—including his medical, mental health and education records, as well as un-redacted state police and law enforcement records. OCA reviewed thousands of pages of documents, consulted with law enforcement and members of the Child Fatality Review Panel, conducted interviews, and incorporated extensive research to develop the report's findings and recommendations.

Key Findings

1. AL presented with significant developmental challenges from earliest childhood, including communication and sensory difficulties, socialization delays, and repetitive behaviors. He was seen by the New Hampshire "Birth to Three" intervention program when he was almost three years old and referred for special education preschool services.
2. The Newtown Public Schools also provided some special education services to AL when he was in elementary school, but services were limited and providers did not identify any communication or social-emotional deficits
3. AL's social-emotional challenges increased after fourth grade.
4. There were early indications of AL's preoccupation with violence, depicted by extremely graphic writings that appeared to have been largely unaddressed by schools and possibly by parents.

5. AL's anxiety began to further impact his ability to attend school and in 8th grade he was placed on "homebound" status through his education plan—a placement for children that are too disabled, even with supports and accommodations, to attend school.

6. AL had several sessions with a community psychiatrist between age 13 and 15, though there are no medical records regarding this physician's treatment. Through brief correspondence with the school the psychiatrist supported Mrs. Lanza's desire to withdraw AL from the school setting in 8th grade.

7. The district provided little surveillance of AL's homebound status, which lasted an entire school year.

8. Recommendations from the Yale Child Study Center, where AL was evaluated at age 14 (AL's 9th grade year), offered prescient observations that withdrawal from school and a strategy of *accommodating* AL, rather than addressing his underlying needs, would lead to a deteriorating life of dysfunction and isolation.

9. Medical and education records reflect repeated reference to AL's diagnosis of Autism Spectrum Disorder, Anxiety, and Obsessive Compulsive Disorder.

10. Records indicate that Mr. Lanza made efforts after the Yale Child Study evaluation to seek treatment, appropriate care coordination, and education planning for AL.

11. Yale's recommendations for extensive special education supports, ongoing expert consultation, and rigorous therapeutic supports embedded into AL's daily life went largely unheeded.

12. AL's resistance to medication recommended for treatment of his Anxiety and Obsessive Compulsive Disorders appeared to be reinforced by his mother. According to records, AL disagreed with his Asperger's diagnosis and may not have understood the benefit of individual therapy.

13. Once AL was diagnosed, AL's education plan did not appropriately classify his disabilities and did not adhere to applicable guidelines regarding education for students with either Autism Spectrum Disorders or Emotional Disturbance.

14. Though AL showed initial progress in 10th grade with the school's plan to incrementally return him to the school environment, his progress was short-lived. By the spring of that year, AL had again withdrawn from most of his classes and had reverted to working on his own or with tutors.

15. AL's parents (and the school) appeared to conceptualize him as intellectually gifted, and much of AL's high school experience catered to his curricular needs. In actuality, psychological testing performed by the school district in high school indicated AL's cognitive abilities were average.

16. AL completed high school through a combination of independent study, tutoring, and classes at a local college.

17. Records indicate that the school system cared about AL's success but also unwittingly enabled Mrs. Lanza's preference to accommodate and appease AL through the educational plan's lack of attention to social-emotional support, failure to provide related services, and agreement to AL's plan of independent study and early graduation at age 17.

18. AL and his parents did not appear to seek or participate in any mental health treatment after 2008. No sustained input from any mental health provider is documented in AL's educational record or medical record after 2006.

19. Though AL was profoundly impaired by anxiety and Obsessive Compulsive Disorder, his parents may not have understood the depth or implications of his disabilities, including his need for ongoing support.

20. AL's pediatric records from age 13 to 17 note his obsessive compulsive behaviors, markedly underweight presentation, psychiatric diagnoses, and repeated homebound or independent study, but records don't clearly address AL's need for mental health treatment, and often note during high school years that no medication or psychiatric treatment was being provided.

21. AL's adult medical records do not reflect awareness or diagnosis of ongoing mental health issues.

22. AL progressively deteriorated in the last years of his life, eventually living in virtual social isolation.

23. AL stopped communicating with his father in 2010 and did not respond to numerous emails Mr. Lanza sent between 2010 and 2012 seeking to spend time with him.

24. AL became increasingly preoccupied with mass murder, encouraged by a cyber-community – a micro society of mass murder enthusiasts with whom he was in email communication.

25. Examination of AL's communications during this time, while suggesting depression and, at times, suicidal ideation, does not suggest the presence of psychosis (loss of contact with reality).

26. AL, who over the years engaged in recreational shooting activities with both of his parents, retained access to numerous firearms and high capacity ammunition magazines even as his mental health deteriorated in late adolescence.

27. In the waning months of AL's life, when his mother noted that he would not leave the house and seemed despondent, it is not clear that any measures were taken to curtail his access to guns or whether the family considered AL's potential for suicide.

28. AL was anorexic at the time of death, measuring 6 feet tall and weighing only 112 pounds. Authors cannot determine what concerns were raised by his mother regarding his eating ability or habits, or his continued emaciation during this time.

29. In the wake of Mrs. Lanza's stated plan to move out of Sandy Hook in 2012, and perhaps stimulated by fears of leaving the "comfort zone" of his home, AL planned and executed the massacre at Sandy Hook Elementary School on December 14, 2012.

30. In the course of AL's entire life, minimal mental health evaluation and treatment (in relation to his apparent need) was obtained. Of the couple of providers that saw AL, only one—the Yale Child Study Center— seemed to appreciate the gravity of AL's presentation, his need for extensive mental health and special education supports, and the critical need for medication to ease his obsessive-compulsive symptoms.

31. This report suggests the role that weaknesses and lapses in the educational and healthcare systems' response and untreated mental illness played in AL's deterioration. *No direct line of causation can be drawn from these to the horrific mass murder at Sandy Hook.*

32. The dynamics presented in this report reflect common concerns over siloed systems of education, physical health, and mental health care for children.

33. Findings in the report strongly implicate the need to assist parents with understanding and addressing the needs of children with complex developmental and mental health disorders.

34. Relevant to this report is that a multi-state review conducted by the federal government confirmed that many states struggle with a dramatic lack of effective services for transition-age youth diagnosed with autism spectrum disorders.

35. While this report focuses on educational, physical and mental health issues, the authors recognize the significant role that assault weapons and high capacity ammunition clips play in mass murder. That AL had ready access to them cannot be ignored as a critical factor in this tragedy. Assault weapons are the single most common denominator in mass shootings in the United States and as such, their ready availability must be considered a critical public health issue.

36. The likelihood of an individual with Autism Spectrum Disorder or severe problems with anxiety and obsessive compulsive tendencies committing an act of pre-meditated violence, much less one of AL's magnitude, is rare. Individuals with those mental health or developmental disorders are more likely to internalize (that is, to feel distressed emotionally or to be confused, socially inappropriate or inept, and sometimes to harm themselves inadvertently or intentionally) than to externalize (that is, to act out aggressively so as to harm others). In AL's case, his severe and deteriorating internalized mental health problems were combined with an atypical preoccupation with violence. Combined with access to deadly weapons, this proved a recipe for mass murder. Autism Spectrum Disorder or other psychiatric problems neither caused nor led to his murderous acts.

37. While authors describe the predisposing factors and compounding stresses in AL's life, *authors do not conclude that they add up to an inevitable arc leading to mass murder.* There is no way to adequately explain why AL was obsessed with mass shootings and how or why he came to act on this obsession. In the end, only he, and he alone, bears responsibility for this monstrous act.

Key Recommendations

Screening

- Systems must facilitate and financially support universal screening for behavioral health and developmental impairments for children ages birth to 21. This is especially necessary within a pediatric primary care setting, with a financial reimbursement strategy to incentivize compliance with screening requirements.

Evaluation

- A child today displaying the types of multidisciplinary developmental challenges AL presented should be referred for thorough evaluation and assessment, including medical, psychological, occupational, speech and language, social-emotional, and neurological testing—evaluation by outside experts should be available to inform clinical and educational decision-making.

Care Coordination and Information Sharing
- Children and their families should have access to quality care coordination, often reserved only for children with complex medical needs, but beneficial for children with developmental challenges and mental health concerns. Care coordination should facilitate more effective information-sharing among medical, community, and educational providers.

Training and Workforce Development
- Teachers, administrators, related service personnel, pediatricians, and parents need access to training and information concerning mental health issues as they arise during the developmental years and in the context of changing environmental expectations.

Support and Engagement with Families
- Providers must have the staffing and financial supports to deliver family-focused support. Services for children and families must be sustained, rather than episodic and periodic. The duration of services must be tied to measurable outcomes rather than predetermined service schedules.
- Effective and sustained family engagement work must be part of mental health treatment for children.
- The role of denial of illness is a relevant theme in this report. While the roots of denial are complex, our healthcare system must address the role that stigma plays in the minimization of psychopathology.
- Parents may be overwhelmed with their own difficulties and the burdens of daily care and support for a youth with significant disabilities. States must increase access to therapeutic services, psycho-education, and peer support for families who have children with specialized needs.
- Systems must be ready to respond supportively and appropriately (up to and including a referral to child protective services) when a parent, even with education and resources, appears unwilling or unable to meet the needs of their child.
- A recurring theme in this report is the struggle of a parent whose child has a severe disability to figure out how to alleviate his pain and protect him from stress and harm. When the parent has difficulties reaching out to helping providers or feels mistrust in the medical and educational systems, her efforts can become unwittingly destructive of the child's development and well-being. Our health care and educational systems must become better at reaching these parents and helping the children.

Education
- The goal of interconnection among separate systems within the mental health arena can only be successfully achieved through the integration of schools and their active participation concerning the mental health and wellness of their students.
- Schools should have support and greater flexibility to retain or import therapeutic and other related services (such as occupational therapy and behaviorist services) into the school setting, and funding and reimbursement mechanisms must be strengthened.

- Schools must ensure that they are evaluating children in all areas of suspected disability, including conducting social-emotional evaluations. This is particularly critical for a student with known or suspected ASD, *even when* academic concerns are neither raised nor immediately evident.

- By asking special education teams to specify a child's eligibility under a specific (or single) label—meaning what is the "right" disability—there is a tendency for interventions to focus on only one aspect of a child's learning and development. This focus on "primary disability" may mitigate against a truly comprehensive support system for the child. It is essential that a more holistic approach to identification for special education eligibility that encourages attention to *multiple* aspects of disability—as was true in AL's case—be undertaken.

- The state/s should consider an audit of existing homebound practices and procedures, and a needs assessment of the population of students who are currently or who have been placed on homebound within a certain timeframe.

- Much more attention needs to be paid to post-secondary readiness for disabled youth and young adults, with a focus not only on academic skills but the ability to live as independently as possible, with or without community supports.

Increase Expertise and Services to Support Children with Developmental and Mental Health Challenges

- A major issue faced by families is the paucity of services and supports for children and youth, particularly older youth and adults, who have Autism Spectrum Disorders with or without co-occurring mental health challenges. State and local educational and mental health and developmental services agencies must work together to identify current capacity and service delivery needs, training opportunities, and must create capacity-building services at all levels.

- Dramatic workforce development needs, increased technical support, and expertise will be required to help mental health, pediatric, and educational providers meaningfully meet the needs of children with complex developmental or mental health disorders, *and their families.*

- Schools may not be equipped to provide, or even to import, comprehensive behavioral health or developmental supports to children, and will need significant support to ensure adequate expertise and related services for children with highly specialized needs.

INTRODUCTION

On Friday, December 14, 2012, our state and nation were rocked by the overwhelming tragedy at Sandy Hook Elementary School; twenty children and six educators were massacred in the school. The gunman committed suicide in one of the classrooms, and his mother lay dead in her bed just a few miles away. More questions than answers reverberated across the nation. From school safety, to gun safety, to mental health treatment, discussions and debates were occurring in all arenas.

On that tragic day, AL age 20, shot and killed his mother Mrs. Lanza, age 52, in their home in Sandy Hook, Connecticut. He shot her four times with a Savage Arms .22 Bolt-Action Long Rifle. He then proceeded to Sandy Hook Elementary School, where he shot his way into the locked building. According to available reports, within 8 minutes the shooter had killed, with an AR-15, twenty children ages 6 & 7, and six school personnel: the school principal, psychologist, teachers, and teachers' assistants. As first responders were nearing the school, AL shot himself with a Glock 20 10mm Auto handgun.

In the immediate aftermath of this indescribable event, state and federal law enforcement agencies began investigating the circumstances leading up to the shooting. The Governor of Connecticut, Dannel Malloy, announced the establishment of the Governor's Sandy Hook Advisory Commission on January 3, 2013, the purpose of which was to "review current policy and make specific recommendations in the areas of public safety, with particular attention paid to school safety, mental health, and gun violence prevention."[1]

On January 30, 2013, the State Child Fatality Review Panel (CFRP) directed the Office of the Child Advocate (OCA) to "begin an investigation regarding the deaths of twenty children at Sandy Hook Elementary School . . . . The investigation would focus on the mechanism(s) that caused the deaths of the children." The CFRP discussed the need for the Office of the Child Advocate to coordinate with other investigating agencies and task forces as well as the need to narrow the scope of the investigation to concentrate on the shooter himself and any systemic recommendations that may emanate from a review of the shooter's history that may support prevention of future tragedies.[2]

---

[1] Press Release, the Office of Governor Dannel Malloy. Gov. Malloy Creates Sandy Hook Advisory Commission to Address Key Policy Areas in Violence Prevention (Jan. 3, 2013), *available at* http://www.governor.ct.gov/malloy/cwp/view.asp?Q=516230&A=4010. Additionally, on January 15, 2013, the Connecticut Legislature created a bipartisan taskforce on gun violence prevention and children's safety. The purpose of the taskforce was to "conduct a review of current law and make recommendations on a range of potential legislation to prevent gun violence, enhance school security and ensure the availability of mental health services in Connecticut." This group looked at school safety and the mental health system. Press releases and recommendations are *available at*: http://www.cga.ct.gov/ASaferConnecticut/.
The Connecticut Legislature also created, via Public Act 13-3, the Behavioral Health Taskforce, charged with reviewing gaps in the state's system for the identification and treatment of adolescents with significant mental health issues. Links to the multi-disciplinary recommendations of the taskforce and a copy of the Public Act are *available at*: http://www.cga.ct.gov/ph/BHTF/taskforce.asp.
[2] The Office of State's Attorney, Judicial District of Danbury also conducted a criminal review and issued a report on November 25, 2013. The purpose of the report was to "identify the person or persons criminally responsible for the twenty-seven homicides that occurred in Newtown, Connecticut, on the morning of December 14, 2012, to determine what crimes were committed, and to indicate if there will be any state prosecutions as a result of the

Statutory Obligations and Authority of the Child Fatality Review Panel and the Connecticut Office of the Child Advocate

The State Child Fatality Review Panel's mandate is outlined by Connecticut General Statute section 46a-13k *et seq*. Specifically, the CFRP "shall review the circumstance of the death of a child placed in out-of-home care or whose death was due to unexpected or unexplained causes to facilitate development of prevention strategies to address identified trends and patterns of risk and to improve coordination of services for children and families in the state."[3] Further, "upon request of two-thirds of the members of the panel . . . or at the Child Advocate's discretion, the Child Advocate *shall conduct an in-depth investigation and review and issue a report* with recommendations on the death or critical incident of a child. The report shall be submitted to the Governor, the General Assembly and to the commissioner of any state agency cited in the report and shall be made available to the general public."[4]

Pursuant to Connecticut General Statute section 46a-13k, the Connecticut Office of the Child Advocate (OCA) has a broad mandate, separate and apart from the Child Fatality Review Panel, to oversee the care and protection of children served by state-funded systems. The statute identifies duties to evaluate the delivery of services to children, review complaints related to children, pursue investigations on behalf of children, review procedures, recommend changes in state polices, take all possible action to ensure the legal, civil, and special rights of children are adhered to, and review the care of children with special needs. OCA also serves as a member and current co-chair of the Child Fatality Review Panel.[5]

OCA holds additional obligations to the General Assembly and the public that require disclosure of findings and recommendations regarding public systems that are determined to be "in the general public interest." The expectation of public disclosure is based upon the expectation of transparency in government and accountability in government performance. Therefore, the report that follows makes public major parts of the documents obtained through the subpoena authority outlined in OCA's statute, for the purpose of informing the public and facilitating a means for follow-up of recommendations. Some information contained in this report may typically be considered confidential. OCA has deep respect for the laws and practice of confidentiality, but pursuant to Connecticut General Statute Sec. 46a-13k *et seq.*, OCA has the authority to disclose confidential information where the interest of a child or the public is affected.

---

incident." OFFICE OF STATE'S ATTORNEY, JUDICIAL DISTRICT OF DANBURY, REPORT OF THE STATE'S ATTORNEY FOR THE JUDICIAL DISTRICT OF DANBURY ON THE SHOOTINGS AT SANDY HOOK ELEMENTARY SCHOOL AND 36 YOGANANDA STREET, NEWTOWN, CONNECTICUT ON DECEMBER 14, 2012 1 (2013), available at http://www.ct.gov/csao/lib/csao/Sandy_Hook_Final_Report.pdf.
[3] Conn. Gen. Stat. §46a-13l(c) (2011).
[4] *Id.* §46a-13l(e) (emphasis added).
[5] OCA was initially established after the tragic homicide of a baby in state child welfare agency custody in 1995. Subsequently, child death review has become an integral component of the OCA enabling statute and a particular focus of the work of the Office. OCA has regularly monitored and reported on child deaths in Connecticut and has prepared and published numerous child death investigative reports for the purpose of informing the public regarding the causes of preventable child death and strategies for prevention.

OCA has determined that it is in the public's interest to acknowledge the strengths and weaknesses of publicly funded child serving systems and promote improvements through a clear picture of the findings and recommendations emanating from this comprehensive fatality review.

Methodology & Documents

Upon completion of the investigation by law enforcement agencies including the State Police and the State's Attorney's Office, Judicial District of Danbury, in December, 2013, the Office of the Child Advocate began a comprehensive collection and review of records related to the life of AL. Using the statutory authority of the Office of the Child Advocate to access information, official records from pediatrics, general health, mental health, education, police, medical examiner, and others were collected as part of this review. All records that were obtained or reviewed were accessed through written requests or issuance of subpoenas. At all times OCA maintained the confidentiality of these records during the review process, including requesting that contributing authors sign confidentiality agreements.

The State Police Report (unredacted) was made available to the OCA as well as specific requests for documents that were part of evidence gathered during the police investigation. OCA reviewed the public report by the State's Attorney, Stephen Sedensky. OCA consulted with a variety of subject matter experts to inform this report, and ultimately sought to co-author the report with the following clinical and educational experts: Harold I. Schwartz, M.D., Julian D. Ford, Ph.D., Andrea Spencer, Ph.D., and Christopher Lyddy, L.C.S.W.

OCA met with families of the children and adults killed in Sandy Hook Elementary School, several of whom expressed an interest in learning more information about the events that led AL to murder their loved ones.

OCA also extended an invitation to meet with Mr. Lanza, the shooter's father, who in the late stages of the report's development provided an extensive interview and private correspondence pertinent to this report. During an interview with OCA, Mr. Lanza was engaged, cooperative, and forthcoming with information he thought would be helpful to authors' analysis of mental health and educational system issues.

Much of OCA's work was done parallel to the work of the Governor's Sandy Hook Advisory Commission. The Sandy Hook Commission, comprised of multiple subcommittees, reviewed and heard testimony from a variety of stakeholders and experts regarding issues including gun safety, school safety and crisis response, neurodevelopmental disorders, mental illness, and law enforcement and emergency response. Two co-authors of this report, Christopher Lyddy, L.C.S.W. and Harold I. Schwartz, M.D., also serve on the Sandy Hook Commission.

OCA consulted with state police investigators, federal law enforcement, the state's attorney's office, and other state officials during the review and development of this report. Authors reviewed dozens of law enforcement interviews of witnesses, persons known to AL, and other relevant parties. State police and federal officials met with hundreds of individuals to fact-find and draw law enforcement conclusions, and the authors of this report did not duplicate this effort. Rather, authors reviewed this material, conducted additional interviews where necessary, and pieced together AL's story to better understand any lessons learned or recommendations for fatality prevention emanating from a review of his circumstances. Despite the breadth of OCA's review, missing pieces of information likely remain, but authors believe that the report represents essential elements of AL's developmental trajectory.

OCA conducted additional research to support expert findings and recommendations regarding early childhood development, best practices for children with neurodevelopmental differences and serious mental health challenges, best practices for pediatrics regarding multidisciplinary assessment and referral, barriers and considerations regarding interagency sharing of confidential health and educational materials, evidence-based methodologies for engaging and providing psycho-education to families of children with significant developmental and mental health challenges, and innovation in service development and delivery for children and adolescents with significant developmental and mental health profiles.

Authors present information in this report by examining AL's life from a chronological perspective, offering findings and recommendations throughout the report. Key documents are also included, for reference, in the appendix to this report.

EARLY YEARS

While it is difficult to imagine AL outside the context of the horrific crime he committed, it was critically important for the authors to understand his story so that authors could identify any important themes that contributed to his mental health deterioration and murderous actions.

AL was born on April 22, 1992 in Exeter, New Hampshire. He lived with his parents, Mrs. Nancy Lanza and Mr. Peter Lanza, and one brother, Ryan, who was older than AL by four years. Mrs. Lanza returned to work after AL's birth for some period of time. Both of Mrs. Lanza and Mr. Lanza's siblings and other extended family members all resided in the greater New Hampshire area.

Mrs. Lanza's pregnancy with AL was reported to be challenging, with maternal hypoglycemia, hypotension, and decreased fetal movement followed by a planned Cesarean section. AL did appear to be a healthy, full-term baby. He apparently had an episode of apnea during which he stopped breathing at eight days old and was admitted to the hospital.

In his early years, AL was described as an extremely active child who did not sleep well, avoided touching, and had early communication problems. He was said to have "made up his own language."

Records indicate concerns about AL's language development in particular. While the authors of this report were not able to obtain a full copy of AL's earliest pediatric records from his time in New Hampshire (birth to five years), his pediatrician appeared to support an evaluation from the state's early intervention system (in Connecticut, referred to as the Birth to Three system) due to AL's speech and language delays. States are required by federal law to offer evaluation and support services for children age birth to thirty-six months who have developmental delays or who have a medical condition that places them at risk for developmental delays.

Authors do not know whether AL underwent any developmental screening by his pediatrician or what concerns his mother or father noted to the doctor during visits. Records indicate that AL underwent a "Birth to Three" evaluation in New Hampshire in late 1994, due to concerns about his communication delays. A pediatric referral was noted in the Birth to Three records. At this time, he was already almost three years old. Birth to Three services end at 36 months.

While it is not unusual for a child to be evaluated by an early intervention provider close to the child's third birthday, in these situations, the evaluation results in recommendations that the family can then use for the child's preschool program. Federal law requires that local school systems have processes for identifying and providing special education and related services for children age 3 to 21 who have a disability that is interfering with the child's education or ability to learn.[6]

The developmental assessment completed by AL's Birth to Three provider indicated that AL "fell well below expectations in social-personal development." The evaluator was unable to understand any of AL's language, needing his mother to serve as an interpreter throughout the testing. Evaluators concluded that AL presented with "significantly delayed development of articulation and expressive language skills."

The evaluation did note that AL had a good attention span, creative play skills, and that he could follow adult directions. The evaluation recommended speech and language services to support communication development and regular pre-school attendance to "stimulate development in all domains."

Because AL was already almost three years old, an initial preschool special education plan was created with recommendations for speech and language support. No other recommended supports or services were noted in the record at this time.

---

[6] Per federal law, school districts are obligated to identify and offer multi-disciplinary evaluation for children who *may* have a disability that is interfering with their ability to make progress in school. 34 C.F.R § 300.304 (2013). A school district's obligations are to pick up where the state's early intervention system leaves off. *Id.* There should be a transition planning meeting from the early intervention system to the local school, and with the participation of the parents and relevant school personnel, a special education plan may be developed. This plan will describe the type of challenges or delays the child presents with, what types of services or supports are required to help the child make progress, and how frequently these services will be delivered. Services may include academic, behavioral or social-emotional, language, occupational, physical, or other supports and therapies. 34 C.F.R § 303.209 (2013).

Pre-School

AL began pre-school in Kingston, New Hampshire in 1995. He attended school several days per week, receiving special education support services, including speech support and occupational therapy as recommended by his Individualized Education Plan (IEP).[7] [8]

It appears from the record that AL was actually removed from speech and language services in late pre-school due to a perception that his challenges were not impeding his ability to learn. Probably as a result of this decision, AL's parents sought an independent evaluation from a local hospital in late April 1997. It appears that as a result of this hospital evaluation, special education supports were reinstated.[9]

The independent evaluation, purportedly a speech and language assessment, showed that AL had several strengths that complemented his developmental challenges. AL was observed to be "friendly [and] bright," with "good social language ability," as well as a good sense of humor. The evaluator posited that AL may have had a sensory integration disorder, and that he displayed "many rituals" in his behavior. Significant speech and language support was recommended in addition to a follow-up with neurology, and work with an occupational therapist certified in sensory integration therapy.

A neurological/developmental evaluation in early April 1997, just before AL's fifth birthday, noted that AL was an extremely active young child—he never slept through the night, continued to make up his own language, and reportedly did not like to be held, kissed or hugged. He was observed and reported to have odd repetitive behaviors and severe temper tantrums.AL was reported, at times, to "sit and hit his head repeatedly." He did not tolerate touch or textures and refused to dress. Teachers reported AL was "very quiet during groups."

---

[7] According to the American Occupational Therapy Association, "occupational therapists and occupational therapy assistants help people across the lifespan participate in the things they want and need to do through the therapeutic use of everyday activities (occupations). Common occupational therapy interventions include helping children with disabilities to participate fully in school and social situations, helping people recovering from injury to regain skills, and providing supports for older adults experiencing physical and cognitive changes." *About Occupational Therapy*, THE AM. OCCUPATIONAL THERAPY ASS'N, INC., http://www.aota.org/About-Occupational-Therapy.aspx (last visited Nov. 3, 2014).

[8] An Individualized Education Plan is the school record which documents the participants in the educational planning process (the IEP team), the primary disability impacting the child, the present levels of the child's performance in various areas of functioning (cognitive, academic, social-emotional), what the goals and objectives will be for learning, how progress will be measured, and what services and supports will be provided to help the child make progress. All supports and services must be research-based or otherwise effective. All decisions for the IEP are made by the team members collectively. 34 C.F.R § 300.321 (2013).

[9] School districts are required by law to consider a parent or guardian's independent evaluation or any other outside assessments and recommendations. The independent reports are not *binding* on the IEP team, but must be reviewed upon the parent's request and may be incorporated into the IEP goals and recommendations. 34 C.F.R § 300.502 (2013).

The school district completed its own developmental assessment in May 1997. The report accompanying the assessment noted that the district had previously decided to discontinue speech supports "because the disability [did] not interfere with educational abilities."[10]

The updated assessment confirmed that AL still had a dramatic discrepancy between expressive and receptive language abilities (a 42 point standard score difference).[11] This meant that AL understood a great deal more than he could communicate and that his ability to make his needs known in a variety of settings was extremely limited or delayed. AL would not or could not speak in groups, and had noted difficulties with auditory memory and auditory processing—meaning he had difficulty taking in auditory information and then great difficulty putting out information.

The school district should have considered the information from the speech and language evaluation and the neurological evaluation conducted in 1997 together, as reported findings were strongly suggestive of autism.

AL's Individualized Education Plan (IEP) provided him with a classification of Speech and Language Impairment and the plan recommended resuming speech and language services, twice weekly, with a focus on improving expressive language and articulation in spontaneous speech.

"Articulation" speaks to how words are formed and spoken, involving the motor aspects of forming words.[12] "Expressive communication" relates to the ability to demonstrate communicative intent.[13] Expressive communication challenges are present when a child cannot find the right words, does not have a developmentally appropriate vocabulary, and cannot put together an appropriate sentence.

An occupational therapy consultation by the school district followed a few months later, in the fall of 1997, noting that AL displayed inconsistent eye contact and scattered motor skills. Though there were reports of seizures in early childhood, records do not indicate whether these were actual epileptic episodes or simply vasovagal (fainting) episodes, or whether they were ever resolved through an in-depth neurological assessment.

AL's developmental and educational history provides important insights into his life experience, none of which *predicted* he would become a mass murderer.

While AL appeared to achieve some developmental milestones within the normal time periods, he had both fine and gross motor delays during preschool years, as well as a number of problems with repetitive behaviors, lack of participation in groups, sensitivity to smells, and intolerance of touch and certain textures. He was observed to hit his head repeatedly.

---

[10] In order for a child to be deemed eligible for special education services he or she must have a disability that is negatively impacting his or her ability to learn.

[11] Such tests have a mean (average) standard score of 100; as such AL's discrepancy is highly significant.

[12] THE SPEECH AND LANGUAGE EVALUATION, COLUMBUS SPEECH AND HEARING CENTER (last visited Nov. 3, 2014), *available at* http://www.columbusspeech.org/speech-and-occupational-therapy/.

[13] *Id.*

The goal of speech therapy, provided as a special education service, was to focus on articulation development and strategies to help AL compensate for the limited intelligibility of his speech when talking with unfamiliar listeners and to improve his ability to talk with peers and adults.

AL did not speak in groups and appeared to be beginning to understand that others could not understand him. He relied on a classmate for communication with others. As noted earlier, a language assessment (CELF-R) showed a very significant differential of scores between expressive and receptive language.

AL was determined eligible for special education with a primary identification of "Oral Expression Disability." He did, however, present with other challenges, including perseverative behaviors, sensory integration challenges, and motor difficulties. While an IEP must identify a child's *primary* area of disability, the law requires that children be evaluated in all areas of suspected disability and be afforded individualized and, where necessary, multidisciplinary supports to help them learn and develop.[14]

In young children with social impairments and restricted and repetitive behaviors, recent studies[15] suggest that expressive communication skills are often associated with social skills for children with autism. Children with expressive language delay are more likely to have social-emotional problems.[16] Put another way, young children who have difficulty communicating may also develop or already exhibit challenges in behavioral or emotional development.

While AL did not have a formal diagnosis of autism in pre-school, despite the findings from his speech/language and neurological evaluations, his behaviors were instead thought to be closely aligned with descriptions of sensory processing disorder by clinicians who evaluated him. Sensory processing disorder is a condition "in which the brain has trouble receiving and responding to information that comes in through the senses."[17] Children with this condition may be oversensitive to things in their environment, with common sounds being painful or overwhelming. Children may also appear hard to engage in conversation or play.[18]

There is disagreement among the professional community as to the existence of sensory processing disorder as a distinct disorder.[19] The symptoms of sensory integration disorder are thought by many to be secondary to other conditions such as autism, anxiety disorder, or attention-deficit disorder. Indeed, the American Academy of Pediatrics has advised against use of the term "sensory processing

[14] 34 C.F.R § 300.304 (2013).
[15] C. Park, et al., *Brief report: The relationship between Language skills, adaptive Behavior and Behavior Problems in Pre-Schoolers with Autism*, 42 JOURNAL OF AUTISM & DEVELOPMENTAL DISORDERS 2761 (2012).
[16] R. C. Tervo, *Language Proficiency, Development, and Behavioral Difficulties in Toddler*, 46 CLINICAL PEDIATRICS 530 (2007).
[17] *Sensory Processing Disorder Treatment*, ASCENT CHILDREN'S HEALTH SERVICES, http://www.ascentchs.com/developmental/sensory-processing (last visited Nov. 3, 2014).
[18] *Id.*
[19] Beth Arky, *The Debate Over Sensory Processing*, CHILD MIND INSTITUTE (July 10, 2013), *available at* http://www.childmind.org/en/posts/articles/debate-over-sensory-processing.

disorder" due to the lack of empirical validation of this construct as a distinct diagnostic entity. Instead, the AAP recognizes that sensory hyper-and hypo-reactivity may be present in a number of different neurodevelopmental disorders.[20]

However, there is research identifying the global nature of sensory processing challenges in autism, and the importance of considering sensory processing problems as a part of the disorder.[21]

The importance of this early evidence of language, social, and sensory processing challenges is also noteworthy because of the research showing a longitudinal relationship between behavioral, emotional, and social difficulties of students with a history of specific language impairment (SLI).[22] It is apparent that early intervention efforts with AL focused on articulation (i.e. the *mechanics* of speech) as the primary concern. While it was clearly the case that AL's speech issues made it difficult for him to be understood, which might well have exacerbated his limited social engagement in pre-school, the larger issue of expressive communication received little attention, as did other aspects of his rituals and sensory sensitivity.

Previous testing indicated that AL's articulation struggles were actually *secondary* to his expressive language disorder. But these particular issues masked the fact that expressive language was extremely delayed in his early education years, and particularly delayed compared to his ability to *understand* language. His delays should have been considered significant for a three-year-old.

Records do not always document the level of services that AL received during these early education years, which professionals were working with him, or the frequency and duration of services. Records do not indicate that AL received a full medical/neurological evaluation, or that he was served by an expert in sensory integration issues.

This appears to have been the start of a pattern of educational evaluation and service delivery that addressed only *aspects* of AL's cognitive and social-emotional development. From early childhood AL never received comprehensive educational assessments that could provide recommendations for cohesive, multidisciplinary supports that took all of his abilities and disabilities into account.

These early descriptors also reflect a pattern of repetitive behaviors and social and communication difficulties that are evident throughout AL's educational history, with the unfortunate consequence of increasing social withdrawal and isolation—less obvious in his years at Sandy Hook Elementary School, but drastically intensifying in middle school and thereafter.

---

[20] American Academy of Pediatrics, *Policy Statement: Sensory Integration Therapies for Children with Developmental and Behavioral Disorders*, 129 J. OF AM. ACAD. OF PEDIATRICS (2012).
[21] J.K. Kern, et al, *Sensory Correlations in Autism*, 11 AUTISM: THE INTERNATIONAL JOURNAL OF RESEARCH & PRACTICE 123 (2007).
[22] M.C. St. Clari, et al., *A Longitudinal Study of Behavioral, Emotional and Social Impairment (SLI)*, 44 JOURNAL OF COMMUNICATION DISORDERS 186 (2011).

SUMMARY AND RECOMMENDATIONS: EARLY YEARS

A review of information regarding AL's early years with his family does not reveal any profound tragedies or traumas. However, records clearly indicate the presence of developmental challenges and opportunities to maximize therapeutic and intensive early intervention.

These observations underscore the importance of parental and pediatric vigilance regarding children's developmental well-being. AL was referred for early intervention late in his toddler years, when he was almost three. By this time, he presented with several developmental challenges, including significant speech and language delays, sensory integration challenges, motor difficulties, and perseverative behaviors.

Children with atypical developmental trajectories or delays often are not referred for an evaluation and services until a pediatrician or parent recognizes that the child is failing to communicate in typical ways. This seems to have been the case with AL. Given the challenges AL presented during the multiple evaluations between ages three and five, he likely displayed developmental delays or difficulties much earlier.

Records indicate that AL's parents worked to secure multiple diagnostic evaluations for him, and that they advocated for specialized services, even going so far as to obtain an independent expert evaluation to ensure that AL would receive appropriate intervention. It is worth noting that while AL's parents sought evaluation for him, neither the parents nor the educational system persevered (or knew to persevere) to ensure that he received neurological follow-up, a comprehensive psychological evaluation, or evaluation of his behavioral and sensory processing challenges. Given the multiple developmental challenges AL exhibited, and the critical importance of early intervention, a more thorough evaluation and ongoing follow-up might have clarified and deepened the understanding of his needs.

Parents are often in the position of recognizing that their child may need help, but not knowing what that help should consist of. Parents are very dependent and necessarily reliant on the recommendations and strategies offered by professionals, from their local pediatrician to specialists and service providers. Parents look to the professionals, including teachers, to know what should be done for their child. Parents may initially trust that these "helping systems" will steer them in the right direction and make the difference for their child. Systems are developed to help facilitate best practices and to serve as a safety net for people who need access to services. When systems aren't created in a way that fosters communication between professionals and families, those systems are left to make ill-informed, albeit well-intentioned, decisions that may miss critical opportunities to help children and their families.

Here, with a child that seemed to need developmental supports, AL's parents may have been optimistic that, with the right expertise and targeted services, he would flourish. Ideally, early diagnostics and intervention will provide information, hope, and help for parents with young children. Emphasis on helping children in *all areas of development* and teaching parents how to best assist their children will maximize learning opportunities for the child and family and set the optimal developmental trajectory.

ADDITIONAL RECOMMENDATIONS FOR EARLY-CHILDHOOD SCREENING, EVALUATION, AND EARLY-INTERVENTION

Routine Developmental and Infant Mental Health Screening

- When evaluations and services are not provided until a child should be speaking and using language, significant opportunity for timely intervention has already passed. Early developmental screening should begin prior to speech onset and should include questions to determine whether a child is struggling with social interactions with others, appropriate use and engagement with toys, nonverbal forms of communication (e.g., pointing, gestures, demonstrating joint attention), behavioral self-regulation, and processing sensory experiences.[23]

- Experts now recommend that infants and toddlers be regularly screened by healthcare providers for developmental and social emotional development. The American Academy of Pediatrics recommends developmental surveillance be a part of each well-child visit, including observations, discussions with parent(s), and documented findings.[24] The AAP also recommends standard screening tools be used during well-child visits at 9, 18, and 24 or 30 months.[25]

- Screening for autism can now be done as early as 18 months and many developmental experts are recommending that such screenings be done by health care providers even earlier in infancy.[26]

- Healthcare payers must facilitate and support universal screening for behavioral health and developmental impairments for children ages birth to 21. This is especially necessary within a pediatric primary care setting, with a financial reimbursement strategy to incentivize compliance with screening requirements.

Support Information Sharing Between Schools, Families, and Educational Providers

- It is essential that critical developmental well-being information be shared between the family, school, and pediatricians to better coordinate information, care, and ensure efficient and quality treatment planning.

- Regular communication between pediatrics and families can bring out parental concerns and assist families and providers with identifying developmental differences and increasing parental understanding of child development.

---

[23] Center for Disease Control and Prevention, KNOW THE SIGNS: ACT EARLY (2014) http://www.cdc.gov/ncbddd/actearly/index.html.

[24] Council on Children With Disabilities, Section on Developmental Behavioral Pediatrics, Bright Futures Steering Committee and Medical Home Initiatives for Children With Special Needs Project Advisory Committee, *Identifying Infants and Young Children with Developmental Disorders in the Medical Home: An Algorithm for Developmental Surveillance and Screening*, 118 **PEDIATRICS** *405–420* (2006)

[25] *Id.*

[26] *Developmental Surveillance and Screening for Autism Spectrum Disorder Guidelines*, AMERICAN ACADEMY OF NEUROLOGY AND THE CHILD NEUROLOGY SOCIETY (Mar. 12, 2014), http://www.cdc.gov/ncbddd/autism/hcp-recommendations.html.

A Note about the Efficacy of Early Evaluations and Intervention

- When formal screening is done by a healthcare provider, rate of referral and connection with early intervention services dramatically increases when compared with the referral rates from pediatricians who rely *solely on observation*.[27]

- With intensive early intervention *prior to age 3*, developmental outcomes improve and impairments may be ameliorated altogether.[28] A longitudinal study of children receiving early intervention services through 36 months indicated that more than 30 percent of these children did not require special education services in kindergarten.[29]

- Broadening access to Birth to Three programs could serve children who are less severely developmentally delayed (many states' current eligibility criteria is 2 standard deviations from the mean in one domain or 1.5 standard deviations from the mean in multiple domains), or who are at risk of impairment.[30] Maximizing opportunities for early intervention is the most efficient and cost-effective way to support positive developmental outcomes for children.

- A child today displaying the types of multidisciplinary developmental challenges AL presented should be referred for thorough evaluation and assessment, including medical, psychological, occupational, speech and language, social-emotional, and neurological testing. An integrated plan should be developed that addresses the needs of the *whole* child, with coordinated care and follow through.

Necessity of Supporting Children in All Areas of Development

- Ensure utilization of appropriate Birth to Three screening or assessment instruments to accurately identify children with mental health problem behavior, and ensure referral to licensed, early childhood mental health providers for a comprehensive diagnostic evaluation. AL's record describes a variety of developmental challenges which go beyond a speech and language or sensory processing problem. A comprehensive diagnostic evaluation, conducted by a psychiatrist, psychologist, or developmental pediatrician, includes assessment of cognitive, emotional, social, and behavioral functioning and can establish a complete and reliable diagnosis of any developmental conditions, including autism. While practice regarding diagnosis and evaluation of children with possible Autism Spectrum Disorders has evolved since AL was first assessed, access to appropriate and *timely* evaluations such as described here often remain a major barrier for families.

- Many of AL's early behavioral difficulties were consistent with a child with sensory integration difficulties. This area of development may be marginalized and not considered

---

[27] SA Rosenberg, et al., *Prevalence of Developmental Delays and Participation in Early Intervention Services for Young Children*, 121 PEDIATRICS E1503–09 (2008); H. Hix-Small, et al., *Impact of Implementing Developmental Screening at 12 and 24 Months in a Pediatric Practice*, 120 PEDIATRICS 381 – 89 (2007).

[28] K. HEBBELER, ET AL., NATIONAL EARLY INTERVENTION LONGITUDINAL STUDY (NEILS), EARLY INTERVENTION FOR INFANTS & TODDLERS WITH DISABILITIES AND THEIR FAMILIES: PARTICIPANTS, SERVICES, AND OUTCOMES (2007), *available at*
http://www.sri.com/neils/pdfs/NEILS_Report_02_07_Final2.pdf

[29] *Id.*

[30] *See* Massachusetts IDEA Part C Program, serving both developmentally delayed and "at-risk" children, thereby maximizing interventions for young children and their children.

until a child is older and showing signs of being on the autism spectrum. However, even children who are not on the autism spectrum, but have attention difficulties or even social-emotional challenges, may struggle with regulating sensory input. [31] Research-based intervention to support improved sensory processing through occupational therapy is a critical service for these children.

- In pre-school, it is essential to recognize the interrelated nature of communication, sensory, and social delays or impairments, as well as cognitive and information-processing deficits. Children require expertly driven assessments and intervention plans. At the pre-school age, addressing one domain of development typically will require integration with other developmental supports.

- States must support communities in expanding the workforce of mental health practitioners and consultants working with early childhood settings. [32]

- States should ensure quality early childhood education, and ensure focus on *social-emotional* as well as cognitive development. This may require using screening tools, use of validated curriculum for social-emotional development, and incorporation of community supports.

ELEMENTARY SCHOOL YEARS

The Lanza family moved to Connecticut in 1998 after Mr. Lanza took a job with General Electric. Emails sent by Mrs. Lanza indicate that she was looking for a "fresh start." The family: Mr. Lanza, Mrs. Lanza, AL, and Ryan, moved to a new home in Sandy Hook.

As early as 1997, there was indication in Mrs. Lanza's medical records that she felt the marriage was having trouble. Mrs. Lanza wrote often to a friend about the long hours Mr. Lanza spent at work. She described Mr. Lanza as often arriving home after AL and Ryan went to bed, and then leaving early the next morning before the children woke. According to Mrs. Lanza, Mr. Lanza was a "workaholic," though she admitted to a close friend that there "were worse things than that."

Mrs. Lanza did not work outside the home at this point, having left her earlier work at an insurance company. Instead, she dedicated her time to homemaking and raising her children. Her emails to friends in 1999 indicated some frustration with or resentment of Mr. Lanza, who she said wanted to work all of the time, do "fun stuff" with the children on weekends, but did not want to be bothered with any "real life" day-to-day troubles.

Mr. Lanza later acknowledged that he was essentially a "weekend father." According to Mrs. Lanza, he took the children on various outings and enjoyed spending time with them. "School activities" kept the family busy, including "plays, concerts, art shows, and picnics." Mrs. Lanza wrote of "Mr. Lanza and the boys going on an overnight camping trip with the cub scouts."

---

[31] J. Owens, J., et al., *Abnormal White Matter Microstructure in Children with Sensory Processing Disorders*, 2 NEURO-IMAGE: CLINICAL 844–53 (2013).
[32] ROBERT WOODS JOHNSON-CHILD TRENDS, ARE THE CHILDREN WELL?: A MODEL AND RECOMMENDATIONS FOR PROMOTING THE MENTAL WELLNESS OF THE NATION'S YOUNG PEOPLE 35 (2014).

Mrs. Lanza also wrote of the busy summers the children had. After AL's fifth-grade year, she wrote that both boys had a full summer planned. They were enrolled in "education connection . . . soccer camp, karate camp, tennis lessons, swimming lessons," and scheduled for visits with relatives and vacation.[33]

Records indicate that Mrs. Lanza and Mr. Lanza separated in 2002, though they did not get divorced until 2009, when AL turned 18.

Social Development during the Elementary School Years

AL was described as being a little "awkward" and developmentally atypical in elementary school. A classmate of AL's later stated:

> AL [was] a nice kid who was sort of withdrawn [though] I could tell he was a little off . . . . AL seemed to get along with everyone, he would interact [with others] but would never engage classmates in conversation. During this school year, I invited all of my classmates over to my house for a birthday party. The one thing that I thought was odd was AL's mother stayed for the entire party.

Mr. Lanza later stated that when AL was 8 or 9 he loved being a kid. Mr. Lanza felt that AL enjoyed being at Sandy Hook Elementary School and that he was "very happy" during this time of his life. A review of records indicates that in some ways AL was or appeared to be socially involved with other children. He participated in school activities, performed in a school play, and attended boy scouts. He played baseball at least two seasons, though he later indicated that he did not like doing this. Authors had few photographs of AL at this time in his life with other children. AL eventually stated during a 2006 psychiatric evaluation (age 14) that he never enjoyed these activities and did them only because his mother wanted him to.

AL appeared to enjoy playing with LEGO toys, and there are pictures and records indicating that Mr. Lanza and AL, or AL and his brother, would construct LEGOs together. AL was described as enjoying Pokémon video games and making up his own games to play. Later in life, video games would take on a larger role as he became increasingly socially isolated in late adolescence. In elementary school, AL was described as being creative, developing strategy games involving maps and characters that he would sometimes play with his father.

AL was 9 when his parents separated in 2002. There was little description in available records regarding his response to his parents' separation, though in a 2006 interview with a child psychiatrist, AL stated that he attributed his parents' divorce to the fact that they must have "irritated" each other as much as they irritated him.

---

[33] Authors did not have records to document or confirm all activities identified here.

The Lanzas shared custody of AL and Ryan, though the children lived primarily with Mrs. Lanza. Mr. Lanza came up often from nearby Stamford, Connecticut to spend time with the children after the separation. He later stated in a 2014 *New Yorker* magazine interview that he did not feel his children were impacted negatively by the separation, because he saw them as often as he did when he lived in the house full time.[34]

Elementary School Education

AL began first grade at Sandy Hook Elementary School in September 1998. Mrs. Lanza's emails stated that she felt AL was initially doing well in school. She wrote that he performed well in first grade and was making friends. By Ryan's later account to police, Sandy Hook Elementary School was AL's life.

AL continued to receive speech and language services and occupational therapy based on the Individual Education Plan (IEP) that was developed in Kingston, New Hampshire.[35] While some teachers in his elementary school reported that he was hesitant or reluctant to participate in the classroom, other adults described him as having appropriate peer relationships and noted that he had made friends since his move to the new school.

In first grade, AL was reported to be reading at grade level and he was determined to be "[a]bove grade level" in math. Educational concerns at this time focused on written expression–attributed to AL's speech delays—an articulation disorder (difficulty with the mechanics of speaking) and weak fine motor skills (using hands and fingers in age-appropriate ways). The issue of a seizure disorder, still unresolved according to available documents, was raised by his mother, but was not seen as a complication. A pediatric visit for joint pain again documented Mrs. Lanza's statements about the potential for seizures if blood was drawn as part of the diagnostic process. The actuality of a seizure disorder remained unclear. Medical records note a history of possible seizure disorder, and a febrile seizure as an infant. One later pediatric record indicates a plan for follow up with an identified pediatric neurologist, but after being contacted, the neurologist indicated that she had no record of AL ever being a patient.

---

[34] Andrew Solomon, *The Reckoning*, THE NEW YORKER (Mar. 17, 2014), *available at* http://www.newyorker.com/magazine/2014/03/17/the-reckoning.

[35] Children are identified as eligible for special education services by an IEP (Individualized Education Plan) team. The team is comprised of school teachers, administrators, an evaluator (possibly the school psychologist), the parent/s or guardian, and other individuals who are necessary for evaluation and planning. Once identified as eligible for special education services, the team will make an individual plan. The plan will outline the individualized supports and modifications that the student requires to make progress in school. The plan is required to address *all aspects of* disability, though a primary disability will be clearly identified. Supports and services must be tailored to the child's needs and must be research-based, or otherwise effective. The key theme of special education law is that the team makes decisions together. The district is responsible for ensuring that plans are created and implemented in a timely fashion, and that all appropriate laws and regulations are followed. If a disagreement about an evaluation or plan cannot be resolved between the guardian and the school district, the law sets out procedures for resolution of any complaint. Ultimately, an independent hearing officer may be asked to resolve an ongoing dispute over a child's education plan.

The IEP team summary from October 1998 indicated that the focus of intervention was for speech and language impairment. AL was to be provided with speech and language support thirty minutes weekly and occupational therapy support 30 minutes weekly. Authors conclude that these durations were minimal and likely inadequate. It is not clear whether the school district was provided, asked for, or considered material from AL's early intervention or preschool program in New Hampshire in planning his current educational program. Best practices would have required such coordination and review.[36]

The educational plan noted concerns regarding AL's written expression (difficulty with spelling due to speech delays), articulation disorder (mechanics of speech), and weak fine motor schools. The record notes that he was "diagnosed" with sensory processing problems, and that the family reported a previous diagnosis of seizure disorder.[37]

AL was described in school records as "respectful" and having appropriate behavior. Teachers also noted, however, that he needed to learn to "take initiative," that he was "timid," and "needed prompting to participate." His IEP included goals to "improve sensory processing related to daily school activities," which would be worked on by exploring tactile sensation without aversive (negative) reactions, focusing on tabletop activities in appropriate ways.

Early in second grade, the occupational therapy was discontinued although he was still having problems with fine motor skills (e.g., shoe-tying and zipping his jacket). Adults continued to describe AL as "conscientious, quiet, but more talkative since he was grouped with another second grade student." He was described as attentive to detail. Teachers reported that sensory processing was improving and that he was no longer distracted by tactile input. An interim report in October described him as an "excellent student and a thoughtful friend to peers" with "wonderful thoughts and ideas to share." Sensory integration goals were removed from AL's IEP. Emphasis remained on improving articulation through speech supports.

By third grade, his speech articulation had improved, although articulation difficulties were still seen to be impacting his ability to make his needs known in the regular classroom setting. During third grade, AL was reportedly "shy" and frequently ill. Records show that he needed to be drawn out in discussion. He was encouraged to participate and share his thoughts in school. There is no reference to repetitive or ritualistic behaviors during this period. An interim report in third grade indicates that AL made a "concerted effort to volunteer answers," but would not ask many questions. His work was "neat and thoughtful" and he was a "good citizen." He would follow rules, help others, and accept responsibility.

---

[36] The IEP from 1998 indicates that previous "records" were reviewed, though specific records or evaluations were not specified.
[37] Authors find no record that is the source for this diagnosis.

AL was deemed to have met all speech goals early in fourth grade and was exited from special education. However, the speech report only indicated that AL had "no error sounds," an observation that did not speak to AL's challenges with expressive language—again a narrow focus on *articulation* as opposed to *communication*.

A brief description in his educational record states that he was performing at age-appropriate levels of academic and social skills. He had met his goal (Level 4) on the Connecticut Mastery Test in Reading, Mathematics, and Writing. The remainder of Grade 4 appears to have been uneventful. But AL continued to have specialized needs that Mrs. Lanza wanted to address. She wrote to Sandy Hook Elementary School on May 18, 2001, looking for careful consideration of his educational plan and selection of a teacher for the upcoming school year:

> AL is a quiet, considerate child with a tendency to withdraw. He has made tremendous strides in your school system and has benefited from speech therapy. He does, however, tend to 'over focus' on rules and can be very hard on himself as a result. This year has been a challenge due, in part, to a slight mismatch in teacher style and student style. I would like to take a moment to praise TEACHER'S recognition of this problem, as well as her efforts to resolve the issue. I realize the difficulty of modifying a classroom approach to accommodate an individual. ANOTHER TEACHER also has been very helpful in keeping AL's stress level at a minimum. I am hoping that next year AL will be placed in a classroom with a more casual feel to it. He responds well to a nurturing environment, and I would like his emphasis to be on learning rather than coping. He focuses on his work, enjoys structure and always adheres to the rules, but a certain level of strictness seems to bring on anxiety and depression. I have appreciated TEACHER'S willingness to work with me on this issue. I believe that if AL is matched to the right environment for his particular learning style, the process could be less teacher-intensive. That would free AL up to enjoy the learning process with a better result for everyone . . . .

The above communication from Mrs. Lanza indicates that despite AL's compliant behavior, she also characterized him as experiencing stress, including depression and anxiety. Mrs. Lanza's note also begins a pattern of attempts to bend or manage the environment for AL, to help him as she put it much later, "get through each day."

Though Mrs. Lanza's communication documents her concerns regarding AL's depression, anxiety, and other social-emotional challenges he might have been having, there is little in his educational record that echoes or responds to Mrs. Lanza's observations.

Social-Emotional Concerns Began to Become More Prominent Later in Elementary School

A present day interview with a family whose child went to school with AL revealed a memory of AL constructing, for a class project, a "hand poem" where he wrote "loser" and "ugly" on his own fingers.

Grade 5 found that AL transitioned from Sandy Hook Elementary to the Reed Intermediate School for Grades 5 and 6. It is not clear whether he transitioned mid-year or at the beginning of the school year. According to school records, he exhibited good effort, made independent application of grade-level concepts and skills, and showed great insight into the motivation of characters in stories he read, as well as solving mathematics problems. He was described as well-liked by his peers and showing appropriate classroom behavior, though his record indicates that he still struggled initiating conversation with anyone.

> Clinical reviewers of this work have noted that the violence depicted far exceeds that typically found in the drawing and creative writing of boys of this age.

"The Big Book of Granny"

While reports were generally positive about AL's conduct and performance in elementary school, he generated and may have submitted, along with another boy in his class who was listed on the "Book" as AL's co-author, an extremely disturbing project in fifth grade called "The Big Book of Granny." The book was spiral-bound with a purple cover, indicating that an adult may have helped him "professionalize" this work. This was a very dramatic text, filled with images and narrative relating child murder, cannibalism, and taxidermy.

According to the present-day statement of the co-author (an individual who as an adult was diagnosed with mental illness and is purportedly living in a residential setting),[38] the book was created following a class assignment to create a comic book-style creative writing project. The co-author claims that the book was bound in school and submitted for a grade. Other reports indicate that AL may have attempted to "sell" the book to peers for 25 cents and that a school administrator spoke to Mrs. Lanza about the matter.[39] There is no clear indication in the educational records that school staff carefully reviewed or were otherwise explicitly aware of the contents. There is no mention in the school record of any staff response to receiving this book or admonishing AL regarding its sale.

The co-author's mother, in a later police interview stated that her child may have written part of this book because he spent a lot of time with AL during this period of time. She told police that AL and her son would do typical boy things together and would ride bikes and play in the neighborhood. AL often spent time at this friend's house and the mother described AL as "normal and polite." Her son had also been to AL's house and had never reported any worries or unusual incidents.

Mrs. Lanza was Concerned Regarding Her Own Health during AL's Youth

A review of Mrs. Lanza's correspondence during AL's early elementary school years indicates that she was frequently preoccupied with what she felt were her potentially serious and possibly terminal health issues.

---

[38] Authors cannot confirm whether this individual is confined involuntarily in a locked setting or whether he is residing in a community-based facility.

[39] Solomon, *supra* note 34, at 6 ("[AL] tried to sell copies of the book at school and got in trouble.").

In the summer of 1999, she wrote often to a friend regarding the "group of [medical] experts" she was seeing, and that she did not think (at the time) she was "going to die." Her letters referenced numerous tests, with alternating optimism about her prognosis and concerns that her "diagnosis is not good" and she may have "limited time left." Mrs. Lanza talked about having had enough time to get [Ryan and AL] settled in, but that she may have only "months to live."

Mrs. Lanza later told a friend that she was diagnosed with a "genetically flawed autoimmune disorder," but that she intended to be discreet about her diagnosis so as to save loved ones "from unnecessary worry." She asked her friend to keep her condition confidential. She continued to write about experiencing seizures, visiting a neurologist and "being tested, and poked, prodded, injected, and tortured."

Mrs. Lanza wrote of additional neurologic problems, telling her friend that she was having "some excruciatingly painful [tests]," and lamenting that her hopes of "any kind of permanent remission [were] gone." Mrs. Lanza wrote that she looked at her boys and worried about what would happen to them. She confided that she had to "put on a big brave face for [her] family," but that in reality she was "terrified." She reported that her doctor warned her that "[her condition] doesn't look good." She urged her friend to celebrate his 40th birthday with gratitude and joy, "thanking God for every year you get to spend with your family."

Despite Mrs. Lanza's preoccupation with her health and concerns about her mortality, a review of her medical records from that time do not confirm a significant neurologic disorder, autoimmune disorder, or multiple sclerosis—the latter a diagnosis she sometimes indicated that she had.

A medical record from her July 1999 neurology follow up indicates that all testing was unremarkable. The record notes that Mrs. Lanza was experiencing "significant stress in her life related to her husband." Additional medical testing was recommended along with "psychotherapy for [Mrs. Lanza's] emotional issues."

Undated typed notes that appear to be crafted by (or with information from) Mrs. Lanza after 2011 indicate that she was diagnosed with MS several years earlier, that it progressed very slowly, and that symptoms had been "at closest, 18 months apart, and at furthest, 4 years apart." Mrs. Lanza indicated that most of her "[s]evere" episodes seemed to happen after surgeries or during "periods of high stress."

In an email from 2009, Mrs. Lanza stated that once she came to terms with her disease, she ultimately decided to keep information about her health quiet. She did not want people treating her like an invalid. She said that she was not in "denial" but that she did not want to "let this thing define me." She said that "one VERY important thing [she] learned . . . [was] to keep a positive attitude and not to dwell on the negative."

There is no indication that Mrs. Lanza was provided a terminal diagnosis by doctors at any time. A 2008 medical record indicates some findings "consistent with [Mrs. Lanza's] known history of multiple sclerosis." A 2010 medical record for AL indicated that there is a "maternal history of [m]ultiple [s]clerosis." However, a 2012 medical record signed by Mrs. Lanza's primary care physician indicated that the physician treated Mrs. Lanza for over eight years, had seen her many times, and had "*never noticed or treated any symptoms of multiple sclerosis.*" The medical form also stated that there were no related medical conditions or history. This medical record was part of an application for insurance. A psychiatric evaluation of AL in October 2006 outlines family medical history but does not identify a history of maternal Multiple Sclerosis, though Mrs. Lanza was present for the evaluation.

During a present-day interview with OCA, Mr. Lanza initially expressed his belief that Mrs. Lanza had been diagnosed with MS in the late 1990's, and that her correspondence from the time likely reflected her emotional state in the wake of her diagnosis. According to Mr. Lanza, she subsequently received periodic treatment and evaluation from that time forward. However, Mr. Lanza then later indicated that, after further review of Mrs. Lanza's records, it did not appear that a doctor seeing Mrs. Lanza in the years prior to her death had actually diagnosed her as having MS, nor did autopsy results confirm the presence of findings consistent with MS.[40]

Authors cannot account for the variable documentation on this issue. However, it is important to note that Mr. Lanza reversed his firm belief in the reliability of Mrs. Lanza's statements regarding her medical condition and treatment following a review of additional relevant documentation. This raises important questions regarding the parents' mutual understanding of the trajectory of AL's educational and mental health treatment, much of which was guided by Mrs. Lanza's interpretation of unfolding events.

SUMMARY AND RECOMMENDATIONS: AGES 5 THROUGH 10

During AL's early elementary school years, Mr. and Mrs. Lanza still lived together in the family home in Sandy Hook. They separated in 2002, AL's fifth grade year. The brothers were described as doing many typical childhood activities. AL was described by some as seeming happy, smiling, and participating in community and school activities.

At the same time, however, more red flags for developmental and mental health concerns remained or emerged. AL began perseverative hand washing, avoiding contact with other people, and becoming increasingly fearful. By fifth grade, AL had written and submitted "The Big Book of Granny"—a significant and violent text—and following that school year, his struggles began to escalate.

Also affecting AL's family life may have been his mother's concern regarding her own health. Authors cannot conclude what may have been at the root of Mrs. Lanza's real or imagined health conditions. But her email correspondences, combined with the lack of substantial findings in the medical records

---

[40] Autopsy information was conveyed by the family to OCA.

suggest a fixation with her health and mortality. How much of this was observable or felt by other members of the family is difficult to conclude and authors cannot speculate. A review of Mrs. Lanza's correspondence however, frequently paints a picture of a woman who seemed preoccupied with anxieties, either about AL or herself. This is a dynamic that continues to be seen as AL moves through adolescence.

It is unclear why AL never received a thorough neurologic evaluation. Despite numerous references to a possible seizure history of seizure disorder, there is no evidence in the pediatric medical records that a follow up evaluation ever took place.

Though AL received some speech support and occupational therapy early on, the frequency and duration of services provided should be considered minimal (half an hour for each service) and likely did not have significant impact for AL's developmental trajectory. AL's services were focused on a very narrow range of behaviors—specific articulation and tolerance for touching instructional materials. AL was then exited from special education services entirely in the fourth grade.

There is no clear indication in the family's records regarding how AL actually socialized or got along with children. Authors note that in early elementary school grades, there is typically one teacher, and classroom activities are structured to support appropriate peer-social interactions. When children transition to upper elementary school and middle school, classes are more specialized, the school environment becomes more complicated, and demands for social and academic independence increase. In other words, the structured nature of the early academic environment may have assisted in stabilizing AL during his earliest years in school, helping him to manage and self-regulate.

For many children with developmental, attention, or social-emotional challenges, middle school eventually becomes a much more difficult transition. Typical adolescent development includes the increasing importance of social interaction and peer groups during the middle school years. Children with Autism or Asperger's Syndrome, who are not demonstrating significant emotional, behavioral, or academic deficits, may sit under other youths' and even other adults' radar. Education plans may not include supports to assist with appropriate socialization and the development of peer relationships.

Most striking during this period of AL's life is the publication and submission of "The Big Book of Granny." There is intense violence featured in this book, and authors conclude that it was not the sort of creation that most children would even know to invent. Mental health professionals contributing to this report determined that the content of "The Big Book of Granny" can only be described as extremely abhorrent and, if it had been carefully reviewed by school staff, it would have suggested the need for a referral to a child psychiatrist or other mental health professional for evaluation. An appropriate evaluation would have required extended discussion with the child about what the book meant and how it came to be written by encouraging extensive elaboration about what the text revealed regarding the child's thoughts and social-emotional processing.

Here, "The Big Book of Granny" suggests that while in many ways AL appeared to be positively developing, by the age of ten, on some level, he was deeply troubled by feelings of rage, hate, and (at least unconscious) murderous impulses. While many children, and especially boys, of this age contend with anger and violent impulses in their play and creative productions, "The Big Book of Granny" stands out, *to mental health professionals,* as a text marked by extreme thoughts of violence that should have signified a need for intervention and evaluation.

There is no evidence of communication in any form between the school and AL's parents about this book. If the book was indeed turned in or otherwise brought to the attention of school officials, there is no indication as to whether its contents were carefully reviewed. The record does not reveal whether the book was carefully reviewed by either of AL's parents, or even whether they would have understood how aberrant the content was from typical youthful creations.

> No direct line can be drawn between a disturbing artistic representation at age 10 and an act of mass violence at age 20.

If the book had been received and carefully considered, professionals could have potentially considered evaluation for a redetermination of special education eligibility.[41] In the context of special education evaluation and eligibility, consideration of the criteria for emotional disturbance would have been appropriate. These criteria include:

- Limited ability to build or maintain satisfactory interpersonal relationships with peers and teachers;
- Inappropriate types of behavior or feelings under normal circumstances;
- A general pervasive mood of unhappiness or depression; and
- A tendency to develop physical symptoms or fears associated with personal or school problems.[42]

It is worth noting that teachers may have limited training or expertise to identify or respond to a student who may be progressing academically but who is also exhibiting difficulties in social emotional development. Teachers may not have a blueprint that tells them how to identify "red flags," when to ask for assessments, or consider further evaluations of children experiencing difficulty with socialization. With today's increased focus on academic achievement and concerns over availability of resources, schools may feel hampered in their efforts to attend to children's overall cognitive and emotional development, despite how necessary this may be for children's ability to learn. Training for teachers, para-educators and administrators—both regular and special education—is essential.

---

[41] A child who has been "exited" from special education services, as AL was after fourth grade, may be re-evaluated and found re-eligible for same or different supports. The district maintains a continuing obligation to "find" all children in the schools who may be operating with a disability that is impacting their ability to learn. Parents maintain a continuing right to raise concerns with district personnel and ask for evaluation and support. 34 C.F.R. 300.111(d) (2013).

[42] 34 C.F.R § 300.7(c)(4) (2013). "Emotional Disturbance" is a category of disability specifically enumerated in the law that may support a determination of a child's eligibility for special education and related services.

Additionally, authors strongly caution that *nothing* in these findings would predict that AL was likely to commit mass murder, even if a better connection had been made between the writing of "The Big Book of Granny" and a need for mental health evaluation and intervention.

What the book does tend to show is a boy who is struggling with disturbing thoughts of extreme violence that seem to have poured out in the form of stories and visual images of a caregiver and child-like character who are alternately victimized by and victimizers of each other. On the surface AL appeared placid (or "neutral" as one teacher later put it), but this book is a clear indication of severe emotional conflict that AL as a 10 year old could not be expected to understand or resolve without help from adults and professionals.

As for his family, again, it must be emphasized how often parents will rely on the judgment of teachers, doctors, and other professionals to guide them as to what their child may need to flourish. This can be true even when the parent feels and believes they know what is in the best interest of their child.

While AL was exited from special education in fourth grade, it is not clear if there were individuals who could recognize the social-emotional red flags in his presentation at school or speak to his family about what kinds of supports might be available either in the school or community to assist him with navigating his social discomfort or other fears.

The goals and objectives from AL's education plan had been primarily focused on articulation, with little recognition of the social aspects of education. An incorrect assumption may have been made that any social isolation AL demonstrated was solely based on the degree of his speech intelligibility. As this difficulty lessened, attention to his social interactions and interpersonal skills also abated.

Today, we know much more than even ten years ago regarding the benefit of supporting children's healthy development from infancy, the value of early intervention, and the connection between communication and social-emotional well-being. Because of our increased knowledge, we have the ability to bring more effective interventions to bear to support children in all aspects of development from an early age. However, in our current educational climate, which critics contend has focused too narrowly on the cognitive achievement of children, with diminishing attention to children's social/emotional, interpersonal, and communication skills, these critical aspects of development may still lack appropriate assessment and intervention.

Moreover, the tendency for school personnel or parents to normalize a child's behavior, particularly when the behavior is not disruptive and the child is not demanding attention in a positive or negative way, is not unusual. Children with emerging social phobias, social communication deficits, and sensory processing issues that limit their ability to interact optimally with other people may stay under the radar at school with parents and teachers waiting for a child to mature, or emerge from his or her shell. It can be a tremendously difficult or painful event for a parent to state or acknowledge "my child may be different," or "my child may need help." The need for things to be "normal" is an understandable dynamic and may be a coping strategy for many caregivers, or even teachers, who have numerous responsibilities to grapple with on a daily basis. But for a parent, however, the effort to suppress his or her own concerns in the hope that things will get better on their own, is a form of denial that can ultimately set in motion a futile and isolating trajectory. In contrast, recognition of the underlying problem and acceptance of the need for information and support provides the pathway to better outcomes for children and their families.

To the extent that AL may have presented to school staff with a high functioning form of autism, it is important to note that these children often go undiagnosed if they are not presenting behavioral challenges or significant distress. If they are bright they will do well on structured assessment instruments and this can mask the extent of their problems. School teams do not typically become concerned about social isolation, attributing it to a shy nature. Thus, AL's inability to start a conversation was noted but overlooked, even though it is a strong indicator of social processing issues. Again, the need for a comprehensive diagnostic evaluation performed by a licensed specialist is evident.

Schools are in a difficult position when confronting these needs. The student is not presenting with marked psychopathology. They are seen as shy, quirky, or anxious, rather than developmentally disabled. School staff do not possess the training to fully understand and diagnose the underlying condition. Teams are understandably reluctant to give as severe a label as autism. Furthermore, as they manage resources, schools may feel constrained to be more conservative with identifying conditions requiring significant special education services.

Additional Recommendations

- Teachers, administrators, related service personnel, pediatricians, and parents need access to training and information concerning mental health issues as they arise during the developmental years and in the context of changing environmental expectations and demands that may intensify stress on emotionally fragile children or children with particular disabilities.
- Teachers also need support for taking the time to get expert consultation and resources must be readily available for teachers so that they can capably individualize support for one child while meeting other classroom needs.
- School personnel, pediatricians, and parents, need ready access to *experts* in children's mental health and developmental conditions, particularly in cases where dramatic evidence emerges suggesting the need for rapid evaluation and recommendations concerning health and safety in school and community settings.
- The State Department of Education should develop and enforce clear guidelines about the need to refer for specialized evaluations of children presenting developmental conditions.
- School records are often fragmentary and not easily accessible for assessment of a developmental chronology. In this case a developmental perspective might have shed light on patterns of increasing isolation and (as evidenced by "The Big Book of Granny") on underlying emotions that are not readily observable within typical classroom routines—especially as the transition from elementary to middle and high school means that creation of a holistic picture of an individual becomes more difficult in departmentalized school schedules. As electronic records have become more prevalent in the medical arena, serious resources should be devoted to creating transportable, comprehensive school records.

- By asking special education teams to specify a child's eligibility under a specific (or single) label—meaning what is the "right" disability—there is a tendency for interventions to focus on only one aspect of a child's learning and development. This focus on "primary disability" may mitigate against a truly comprehensive support system for the child. It is essential that a more holistic approach to identification for special education eligibility that encourages attention to *multiple* aspects of disability—as was true in AL's case—be undertaken.

AGES 11 THROUGH 14

In a later police interview, Mr. Lanza noted that when AL was between the ages of 11 and 12, he began to seem a little different, less happy. To Mr. Lanza, AL grew more anxious and frustrated, though he did not seem to Mr. Lanza to be angry or aggressive. He didn't like to be photographed or seen in pictures. AL had trouble concentrating and seemed easily overloaded. He began avoiding eye contact and became increasingly anxious. Mr. Lanza reported that AL experienced panic attacks that compelled his mother to come to school.[43]

A parent in the neighborhood later described AL:

> [He was] not connecting with anyone at all . . . he was not bullied, however, he
> was just left alone . . . he never associated with others and when he got on the
> bus he would sit with his headphones and listen to music. [My daughter] tried
> to be nice by saying hi, but AL would not make eye contact with others.

The neighbor invited the family over for Christmas Eve over the years, but they "only came once." Mrs. Lanza however "came to [neighbor's] home several times and seemed convinced AL was sick." Despite AL's increasing anxiety and withdrawal, Grade 6 continued his positive academic trend, with A's and B's across content areas. In an interview with the state police, a teacher at Reed Intermediate School remembered him as bright, if reluctant, with good ideas regarding creative writing. AL would not necessarily engage in conversation, but he would not ignore others. This teacher remembered no incidents of bullying or teasing, a common refrain from virtually all teachers or other former classmates of AL's. Another teacher who had worked with him from 2002–04 remembered him as a shy, quiet boy who listened and participated in class. His demeanor was described as "neutral" most of the time.

During the same time period a pediatric record (2003) noted obsessive-compulsive tendencies, including hand washing, leading to excoriated skin, and clothing rituals. There is no documentation in the pediatric record of any exploration of these issues or of a referral to a mental health specialist.

AL attended Newtown Middle School for grade 7. It was during Grade 7 that his social, emotional, and communicative struggles appeared to have become increasingly intense, culminating in his abrupt withdrawal from the Newtown Middle School at the end of the third quarter, in late April 2005. There is no indication in the record that he was offered a re-evaluation for special education services based on social-emotional or other developmental concerns.

---

[43] Solomon, *supra* note 34, at 9.

There is no information concerning the reason for AL's abrupt withdrawal from school—or the subsequent enrollment in a catholic school—except for a later reference in a psychological evaluation conducted by the Newtown Public School psychologist in 2006, when AL was 14 years old. The district's review indicated that AL began having extreme difficulty in middle school, though these difficulties are not spelled out in detail and there is no reference to a comprehensive plan to address them at the time of his withdrawal. Given the circumstances of his withdrawal from school, it would have been appropriate for these concerns to have been considered in the 2006 psychological evaluation conducted by district personnel, and a subsequent plan developed to address the difficulty noted in the district's review.

Transfer to Catholic School

AL's mother transferred him to a local catholic school for the fourth quarter of 7th grade. Later reports indicate that he "became obsessed with religion,"[44] though there is nothing in the catholic school's record regarding this development. A teacher at the school later reported that he presented very differently from the other children.

> [A]fter my years of experience teaching 7th grade boys, I know how they are supposed to act. But I saw AL as being not normal with very distinct anti-social issues. AL was a very intelligent boy but he was also very quiet, barely spoke, and never responded to his classmates' kindness of trying to help him fit in . . . . I also remember AL never wanting to participate in anything . . . . I truly do not believe that AL's parents were upfront with teachers about AL's mental capacities . . . . I remember giving creative writing assignments to students, instructing them to write a page or two on whatever they wanted to talk about . . . AL would write ten pages obsessing about battles, destruction and war.

> I have known 7th grade boys to talk about things like this, but AL's level of violence was disturbing. I remember showing the writings to the principal at the time, AL's creative writing was so graphic that it could not be shared.[45]

There is no documentation that teachers explored the source of the violent content of his writings with AL or his parents. There is also no indication that Mr. or Mrs. Lanza were aware or were reviewing what AL was producing for school, or whether they had any concerns about it at all. The teacher indicated that she asked AL to write something non-violent for a presentation to parents, and she noted that he was able to produce this alternative writing.

---

[44] A subsequent psychological evaluation conducted by the public school system indicated that AL became obsessed with religion while attending catholic school. The source for this information is not clear. The Yale Child Study Center psychiatrist's report (*see infra*) in 2006 states that "AL disapproves of religion because it is 'illogical' . . . [which] proved the downfall of a brief placement at a small supportive Catholic parochial school."
[45] There is no copy in the educational record of this disturbed writing.

> I remember instructing AL that he had to write something else to share . . .
> [so] instead he wrote a poem that from what I recall was beautiful. AL shared
> his poem in public with his father present who was in tears. I believe his father
> was in tears because he never heard AL recite anything that nice before and
> the surprising fact was that he was able to deliver the poem in public. At the
> end of the school year, I remember AL leaving abruptly . . . .

As the teacher described above, AL was withdrawn from the catholic school by his family at the end of the year and kept at home for a period of time. There is no information about his admission to, or performance at, the catholic school other than his seventh grade report card, which reported solid academic performance. Though AL did not return to catholic school, records indicated that he wanted to keep wearing his school uniform for a time. He did not return to school, public or private, in eighth grade.

AL's Mother Takes Him to the Danbury Emergency Room: September 2005 (8TH Grade)

In September 2005—AL's 8th grade year—Mrs. Lanza took him to the Emergency Room of Danbury Hospital for a crisis evaluation. Mrs. Lanza described AL to health care providers as having had "borderline autism" in the past, but having since outgrown it. She reported that AL was having trouble in school, trouble in groups, and exhibiting repetitive behaviors which had gotten worse in recent days. Mother reportedly feared the "beginning of possible autism." Mrs. Lanza did not believe AL was on drugs, homicidal, or suicidal.

Hospital records described him as "anxious," "withdrawn," and "hesitant to be touched." He presented as agitated, hyper-vigilant, and overwhelmed with fear. The clinical consultation resulted in diagnoses of Anxiety Disorder, NOS;[46] Rule out Asperger Syndrome; Rule out Autistic Disorder, followed by a discharge diagnosis of Asperger Syndrome and Obsessive Compulsive Disorder.[47]

Mrs. Lanza declined an extensive medical work up for AL, indicating that he was already scheduled to see a psychiatrist in three weeks. AL was evaluated by the hospital crisis team and recommendations for therapeutic support were discussed with Mrs. Lanza. The hospital recommended additional evaluation by staff psychiatry. Mrs. Lanza declined this recommendation, stating that AL would be "better off" at home rather than staying at the hospital for further work-up. Mrs. Lanza thought that she could manage him at home and that he was not at risk or a danger to himself or others. Mrs. Lanza stated that she wanted to get him home because he was "very comfortable" at home and would not be as anxious.

Though Mrs. Lanza told hospital personnel that her sole reason for taking AL to the emergency room was to obtain medical permission to allow him to stay home from school indefinitely, the clinical

---

[46] Not Otherwise Specified.

[47] Asperger Syndrome and Autistic Spectrum Disorder were separate diagnoses in the DSM 4 but are now considered variants of the same diagnosis in the DSM 5. Johnson Center for Child Health and Development, *Updates to the APA in DSM-V – What Do the Changes Mean to Families Living with Autism?*, AUTISM RESEARCH INSTITUTE, http://www.autism.com/news_dsmV (last visited Nov. 3, 2014).

team at Danbury Hospital provided information to her regarding next steps for evaluation and treatment. Hospital staff recommended a therapeutic educational placement at the Center for Child and Adolescent Treatment Services (CCATS), and the hospital offered a full evaluation of him to expedite admission to the school.

Mrs. Lanza declined the additional evaluation and referral as documented by the clinical team at Danbury Hospital. She requested that the hospital issue a note excusing AL from school due to the stress level it created for him. Hospital staff agreed to provide a note excusing AL from school for *three days*, pending an IEP meeting. Mrs. Lanza agreed in writing to return him to the Emergency Department should his anxiety symptoms increase at home. The hospital agreed to discharge AL. It does not appear that a subsequent IEP meeting took place until December 2005.

Treatment by a Community Psychiatrist: Beginning Fall 2005

After the Danbury Hospital emergency visit, AL began seeing a local psychiatrist. While there is no indication in available records how Mrs. Lanza identified or connected AL with a community psychiatrist, a former Newtown school official reported having referred Mrs. Lanza to this psychiatrist.[48]

The community psychiatrist later stated that Mrs. Lanza was not interested in having AL take medication to ameliorate any of his symptoms. The community psychiatrist remembered having conversations with Mrs. Lanza and meeting AL (or sometimes both AL and his mother) for appointments. Present day telephone interviews with the community psychiatrist revealed that AL's medical records were, at some point, destroyed. There were, therefore, no treatment records available to review other than some correspondence between the community psychiatrist and AL's school, dated 2005 and 2006. There were no copies of this psychiatrist's evaluation or treatment of AL contained in AL's pediatrician's records, and no copies found by authors in state police evidence files from the Lanza home.

Available billing records documented at least 20 payments to the community psychiatrist by AL's family between November 15, 2005 and July, 2007, with one payment in October, 2008. There was

---

[48] While a school official did share this recollection with OCA interviewers, authors cannot independently confirm this recollection, and other records indicate Mrs. Lanza may have already had an appointment with the community psychiatrist set up at the time of the Danbury Hospital emergency department visit. Staff from OCA spoke with this psychiatrist during the course of this investigation in an effort to identify and obtain records related to the doctor's evaluation and treatment of AL. The doctor indicated that all treatment records were destroyed. Invoices related to provision of treatment by this psychiatrist were contained in evidence recovered from the Lanza home by state police. Records indicate that individual psychotherapy and medication management were billed by the community psychiatrist at least from October 2005 through December 2006. Copies of billing records obtained and reviewed by OCA may not constitute the universe of billing record available. Extensive documentation related to AL's medical history and the interview with the psychiatrist indicate that at no time did AL agree to the community psychiatrist's recommendation for medication. The psychiatrist subsequently and voluntarily surrendered his license to practice in both Connecticut and New York following multiple allegations of sexual relationships or sexual behavior with clients. Josh Kovner, *Lanza's Psychiatrist Later Surrendered License After "Sexual Relationship" With Patient*, HARTFORD COURANT (Dec. 30, 2012), *available at* http://articles.courant.com/2013-12-30/news/hc-paul-fox-misconduct-1230-20131229_1_adam-lanza-female-patient-fox.

also a bill for consulting with AL's IEP team in December, 2005.[49] Establishing the timing and duration of the psychiatrist's clinical relationship with AL is important, given that school records contain scant documentation regarding this psychiatric treatment past early 2006 and educational plans beyond that time do not document input from any mental health professionals.

In a phone interview with OCA staff conducted in August 2013, this psychiatrist initially had trouble recalling AL, then remembered that he had Asperger's Syndrome, that AL and his mother were resistant to medication, that he saw Mrs. Lanza 1 or 2 times alone, and saw AL approximately 8 times. Records obtained by OCA provide a picture of a longer and more extensive relationship between the community psychiatrist and AL than portrayed by this psychiatrist in multiple interviews.

However, the extent of AL's actual participation with or progress in treatment or what treatment actually was provided cannot be confirmed due to the psychiatrist's lack of records, and the absence of any meaningful corroboration of the treatment, including the lack of any treatment records or recommendations in the pediatric or educational file for the bulk of this time period.

Medical Records

In 2003, the pediatric record indicates that AL was 11 years old and had "obsessive compulsive tendencies" such as repetitive hand washing and shirt pulling. He was noted to have excoriated areas on his hands. He was prescribed Aquaphor, an over-the-counter skin care ointment, due to "obsessive washing behavior." There are no documented referrals in the pediatric medical record for counseling, evaluation, or treatment of any underlying condition leading to these behaviors.

There were no documented well-child visits between 11/24/03 and 9/11/06. In 2005 AL had numerous sick visits for sore throats, difficulty breathing, and marked weight loss. There is no documentation regarding follow up blood work or other evaluations to examine underlying causes for these symptoms, particularly the weight loss.

On September 19, 2005, days before AL was seen for crisis evaluation at Danbury Hospital, the medical record notes parental concerns regarding AL not sleeping well, not eating well, and "sleeping a lot during the day." The same record notes that his weight had dropped to 98 pounds. He was approximately 5 feet, 8 inches at that time.

The pediatric record documents AL's trip to the Danbury Hospital emergency department in September 2005 and Mrs. Lanza's request for a note for school given AL's extreme anxiety. The pediatrician's record later indicates that AL and his mother walked out of the emergency room because the crisis center made AL more anxious. Mrs. Lanza was provided with a 3 day "excuse note" for school by Danbury Hospital. It appears that Mrs. Lanza may then have sought a longer excuse note from the pediatrician, pending AL's October visit with the community psychiatrist. As further

---

[49]In a phone interview between the community psychiatrist and OCA, the psychiatrist also indicated that he saw AL approximately 8 times. In a police interview, the psychiatrist indicated that he saw AL when he was about age 15.

outlined below, the psychiatrist then immediately penned the indefinite excuse note sought by Mrs. Lanza. It does not appear that AL was seen again by the pediatrician until June the following year.

A present-day interview with a former school district administrator reveals that, at some point subsequent to AL's emergency department visit Mrs. Lanza visited the administrator in her district office and indicated her desire to "home school" AL. Mrs. Lanza recounted her visit with AL to the emergency department and her concerns regarding AL's anxiety. The administrator remembered that Mrs. Lanza said she had to take AL back home because he was so anxious in the emergency department that it felt "abusive" to keep him there. The administrator did not feel it would be appropriate to home school AL, and instead recommended that the family and school work together to try and meet AL's needs, even in unconventional ways if necessary.

Education: Homebound

Though in September 2005, Danbury Hospital staff gave mother a note excusing AL from school for only three days, the community psychiatrist, upon initial evaluation of AL, only weeks later immediately penned a letter stating that AL should "not attend school due to the lack of an appropriate placement" and his "mounting overwhelming anxiety."

It is not clear what caused the community psychiatrist to opine that there was no appropriate educational placement. There is no indication as to whether Mrs. Lanza shared Danbury Hospital's recommendations for therapeutic school placement with the community psychiatrist or the IEP team. There is no indication in available treatment or education records that the issue of school placement, therapeutic or otherwise, had ever been explored or even discussed with the school district. Therefore, this statement of the psychiatrist is difficult to interpret. Even more curious was his statement in the same correspondence to district officials:

> [AL] has agreed to achieve competency in all academic subjects at home. At this point tutoring is not needed and could be viewed as counter- productive both academically and emotionally.

Clinical and educational professionals contributing to this report agree that the recommendations articulated here by the community psychiatrist were completely inappropriate and non-therapeutic for AL. In subsequent correspondence with Newtown Public School personnel, the community psychiatrist referred to evaluations he had conducted of AL in September, October, and November 2005 that led to his conclusion that AL had Asperger's Syndrome. Again, he recommended that AL be excused from attending school indefinitely:[50]

> AL is a 13 year old boy who I have evaluated on 9/30/05, 10/18/05, and 11/15/05. He meets the DSM IV criteria for Asperger's Disorder. AL presents with a significant social impairment including lack of peer relationships,

---

[50] See accompanying Appendix for Connecticut regulation applicable to homebound instruction, operative through 2013.

avoidance of eye to eye gaze, lack of understanding of how to play or interact with peers. He avoids peer interaction and is very anxious around strangers. He lacks empathy and tends to employ a very rigid systematic thought process. He demonstrates intense emotional rage when his systematic world is threatened due to his extreme need for routine. He tends to take a very literal interpretation of written and verbal material. Concepts like metaphor, symbolism and intangible references are exceedingly difficult for him and can cause significant distress. He tends to have an overly precise quality of speech and tends to not comprehend emotional expression in others. He is phobic [of] physical contact, even with his own mother who has been his most constant and consistent individual in his life.

Due to his extreme anxiety and emotional discord due to minor changes in routines and/or his expectations he is unable to attend school.

Due to his need for systematic precision and logic there needs to be modifications in the school curriculum. For example, the English curriculum should focus on the grammar and writing in a clear precise way. Literary choices should tend to be more literal and less figurative. It would be constructive for AL to have an accelerated program in Math and Science by allowing him to take honor classes in the high school.

At this point I am strongly recommending that AL not be compelled to attend school. He has clearly demonstrated that the experience of the school setting which has an intolerable level of noise and unpredictable elements would promote extreme anxiety and discomfort.

If you have any questions please do not hesitate to call.

The school district followed up on the psychiatrist's recommendations at an IEP meeting in December 2005 with an offer to evaluate AL.[51] This recommendation was declined by Mrs. Lanza, who stated that evaluations at that time would "not be in [AL's] best interests." The IEP indicated that AL was to receive up to 10 hours of special education in the form of tutoring based on the psychiatrist's belief that AL could not function in a regular education environment.[52] There is no documentation that the IEP team considered any potential detrimental effects of this home-bound placement for AL, one of the most restrictive alternative educational options.

There is no copy of any evaluation or treatment recommendations from the community psychiatrist in the school record, though he was present for this meeting. The psychiatrist's formal recommendations in a written report should have been required at this time.

---

[51] Here it appears that AL was being re-evaluated for the purpose of determining special education eligibility, primary disability, and what supports and services will be needed.
[52] AL was placed on homebound status, a "placement" permitted when a child's disability precludes them from being in school, even with provision of individualized modifications and supports. 34 C.F.R. § 300.115 (2013); Conn. Gen. Stat. § 10-76d-15 (2013).

The educational record indicates that potential evaluators would begin to meet with AL as tutoring progressed to try to establish rapport with him. There is no evidence regarding how or if the recommended 10 hours per week of homebound instruction was delivered during this school year. Frequent service delivery would have provided an opportunity for school personnel to observe AL directly in his most familiar setting, and at a time when he was more severely withdrawn and isolated. Better supervision or oversight by the district to patterns regarding homebound service delivery could have triggered added understanding of AL and his needs, with a subsequent reconvening of the IEP team to discuss additional necessary supports or the need for treatment. AL maintained enrollment in school during these times.

For the next several months, AL remained home with his mother. Records indicate that AL may have received tutoring from both his mother and father each week. In March 2006, the psychiatrist responded to a request for information from the school district regarding AL's availability for standardized testing.

The school district sent a note to the psychiatrist stating:

> In order to exempt [AL] from taking the CMTS, we need a letter from you indicating that he is unable to attend school and is medically/emotionally unavailable for homebound instruction for the testing period and the make-up testing period . . . without this letter, we are mandated to send a certified teacher to [AL]'s house to give him the test.

The psychiatrist responded with a faxed note that AL was "medically/emotionally unavailable to be tested (CMT)." According to the psychiatrist, AL could not and *was not receiving home-bound or hospital-based tutoring and he was not attending school at all.*

A June 2006 IEP record noted that AL's primary disability was "to be determined,"[53] but the team agreed to defer evaluation due to his extreme anxiety and the psychiatrist's recommendations. A schedule of courses was listed for his possible 9th grade entry into Newtown High School.

A Note about Home-Bound Educational Placement versus Homeschooling

AL was not "homeschooled." He was initially informally withdrawn from school by his family, provided a medical "excuse note," and then via the special education planning process his IEP team agreed to a recommendation that he would be placed on *homebound* status. *Homebound* status is permitted by Connecticut education law when a child is deemed too disabled to receive services in school even with modifications and supports.[54] For a child who is identified as eligible for special education services, the school district must provide instruction in the home so that the child can

---

[53] The IEP team could have, at this point, identified AL's primary disability as Autism or Emotional Disturbance based on his diagnoses from the community psychiatrist.
[54] REGS. OF CT. STATE AGENCIES, § 10-76d-15 (2013) (regulations operative during AL's high school years are included in the Appendix to this report).

maintain the continuity of his school program.[55] The new IEP approving homebound placement must indicate what the instructional objectives will be in the restrictive setting. For an IEP team to approve homebound instruction, there must be a physician's note that the child cannot go to school (with an expected date when the child could return). The recommendation must specify the severity of the child's challenges or document that his or her presence endangers other children.

> **Homebound status is considered the most restrictive setting for a child's education.**

Home-schooling, by distinction, is an option exercised by a parent who wishes to provide instruction to a child in the home or community that is, at minimum, equivalent to education provided in the public school setting.[56]

Connecticut law requires parents and guardians to ensure that their children are instructed "in reading, writing, spelling, English grammar, geography, arithmetic and United States history and in citizenship, including a study of the town, state and federal governments."[57] Enrollment of a school-age child is considered mandatory unless the guardian "is able to show that the child is elsewhere receiving equivalent instruction in the studies taught in the public schools."[58]

Where a child is "homeschooled," as opposed to "homebound status" via an IEP, the local school district is not required to provide any special education services.

Here, it appears that AL's family sought to have him placed on homebound status and the family provided a doctor's note to support this recommendation. Although AL was entitled to receive up to ten hours per week of tutoring from the school district and to work towards the goals in his IEP, at certain times all educational supports from the district were refused. It is not evidenced that these hours were provided, or how many home visits or hours were refused and why.

SUMMARY AND RECOMMENDATIONS: AGES 11 THROUGH 14

AL's mental health began to significantly deteriorate during middle school. His family noticed his anxiety increasing, his pediatric record notes emerging obsessive-compulsive behaviors, and he began to struggle with attending school. His family, looking for solutions to help AL and perhaps lacking expert advice, responded to these challenges by changing his environment, moving him from one school to another, and then withdrawing him and allowing him to stay home. This began a pattern of enrollment and withdrawal that culminated with AL's later retreat from high school and ultimate isolation from the community post-graduation.

While there is a body of evidence showing that AL's anxiety increased over these years, there is no clear indication of why this happened. For children with autism, this pattern often occurs in the face of escalating academic, social, and adaptive demands with which they cannot keep up. There is also a high risk of bullying or mistreatment by peers which can lead to this type of reaction in late elementary school or middle school, though there is no evidence in AL's record to support a finding

---

[55]*Id.*
[56]CONN. GEN. STAT. § 10-184 (2014).
[57] *Id.*
[58] *Id.*

he was bullied. Something was occurring (developmentally, in the family, or in the school) that was fueling the regression and the family's efforts to take him out of the school programs.

Mrs. Lanza appears to have gone to three health care providers to obtain an "[e]xcuse note" that she sought for AL. It is never clear that the Lanzas understood the detrimental effects of enabling AL's isolation from the community and peers, at least at this time.

Up until this point, no one, other than the health care providers at Danbury Hospital, appeared to educate the Lanzas about the potential harms of extended homebound status or school withdrawal, or provide meaningful alternatives for treatment and education. In an interview with journalist Andrew Solomon, Mr. Lanza reported that he felt some relief at AL's diagnosis of Asperger's Syndrome and that he researched options for education, including private schools.[59] Mr. Lanza indicated that he went to a meeting of the Global and Regional Asperger Syndrome Partnership to see what options existed in the world for his son.[60]

It is necessary to consider how the community systems of care: the Emergency Department, pediatrician, school system—intersected with this family. What role should AL's pediatrician have played in assessing AL's mental health and connecting him and his parents to appropriate supports in the community or in helping them identify the nature and extent of AL's disabilities? There does not appear to be any follow up to 2003 observation of compulsive behavior that led to significant hand excoriation and irritation—no referrals for mental health evaluation or treatment. As stated above, there is little follow-up in the medical record after AL's visit to Danbury Hospital or with regard to his treatment by the community psychiatrist.

The scant documentation regarding these important matters appears to continue despite the notation in the pediatric record that AL was being "home schooled" due to his extreme anxiety and AL's pattern of concerning medical complaints regarding eating difficulties, weight loss, and breathing problems. At one point he was prescribed both Aquaphor for excoriated hands and later (after 2006) Miralax for constipation, yet there appears to be little attention for ongoing mental health evaluation and treatment, and no documentation of correspondence or coordination of care between the pediatrician and the treating psychiatrist. Additionally, there is nothing in the record to indicate that the pediatrician observed or referred Mr. or Mrs. Lanza for family counseling. It appears, at least from what is documented in the medical record, that the pediatrician's approach to AL was similar to that of the school and the family: management of AL's peripheral symptoms rather than actual thorough evaluation and treatment of the underlying challenges affecting him or his family.

What response could the school system have had, and what was its capacity to screen and evaluate AL in all areas of suspected disability, as required by state and federal law? The school district appears to have accepted the recommendations of the mother and the community psychiatrist for homebound placement (without instruction) with no documented discussion of alternatives. It is

---

[59] Solomon, *supra* note 34, at 9.
[60] *Id.*

difficult to determine why there was no review of therapeutic school settings as a consideration for placement or even other therapeutic supports that could be put in place for AL in the school setting. Additionally, there was very little scrutiny of AL's homebound placement.

In October 2005, the school first received the community psychiatrist's note that AL could not come to school due to anxiety. But the district did not convene an IEP meeting until December 2005, at which time the homebound status was confirmed and extended. March, 2006 saw the school district reach out to the psychiatrist, but only to review AL's availability for standardized testing. There did not appear to be any significant or timely follow up to the psychiatrist's reply that AL was not only unavailable for testing, but unavailable for *any instruction whatsoever*.

The IEP team did not reconvene until June, 2006 to discuss the upcoming school year. Though there was a release of information signed by Mrs. Lanza that permitted the school district to discuss AL with the community psychiatrist, there is no documentation in the school record that the district had a treatment plan for him, or that the district raised any questions about AL being out of the school for an entire year. State regulations permit not only homebound instruction, but also hospitalized instruction. In the face of disabilities that were so significant as to apparently justify AL's lack of attendance for the entire school year it does not appear that anyone questioned why, if he was so debilitated, he was never hospitalized or referred for specialized educational placement. On a number of levels and on numerous occasions, the district did not follow appropriate procedures, monitor AL's IEP progress for goals and objectives, or document attempts to follow up with providers or the family regarding psychiatric or pediatric care.

As for the local hospital where AL was seen in the emergency room in 2005, it appears that hospital personnel immediately identified him as a youth with potentially significant mental health needs. The recommendations made by the hospital for psychiatric evaluation, follow up, educational planning, and possible placement in a therapeutic school setting, all appear sound and appropriate.

Confidentiality laws do not permit the hospital to share medical records without the express consent of the family. Given this privilege, the Lanzas were the legal gatekeeper for sharing available information. It is not clear, however, whether the hospital sought to have the parent sign a release to share their observations and recommendations with the school district or the community psychiatrist, but the record does not document that this request was made or declined. Here, the hospital was told that Mrs. Lanza was following up with a community psychiatrist in just a couple of weeks. It appears that health care professionals reluctantly concluded that AL could hang on until then.

Our health care system is grappling now with the role that various community institutions should or must play in assisting with the identification of children with special health care needs, engagement with families and referral to appropriate and effective supports. A true model for children's wellness must promote integration between community service systems, ease of information sharing between pediatrics, families, and schools, and recognition that

> The lack of an effective system, or capacity, for information-sharing and care coordination between providers, family and school, is a critical theme in this report.

children's wellbeing is about healthy growth in *all* areas of development—cognitive, social-emotional, and physical.

Even today our children's services system suffers from a siloed approach, where one provider may know little about the recommendations of another. In AL's case, Emergency Department staff may not have been in a position at the time of his visit to doubt or compel the family's follow up, or to communicate with the school without Mrs. Lanza's approval. The community psychiatrist ultimately made drastically different recommendations than the Emergency Department staff, and these were the recommendations that were provided to and adopted by the school system.

Homebound Students

Records confirm that AL was placed on homebound status beginning in 8th grade and, at times, his family declined all district supports, including tutoring. Although an initial doctor's note was provided recommending homebound placement and refusing tutoring, records show that there was little oversight of this placement or any meaningful consideration of alternatives. AL remained on homebound status for a long period of time without documentation that he was seeing or receiving treatment. His IEP team, which included his family, did not revisit what therapeutic supports he might need to be returned to a school setting. At this time, the Lanzas may well have relied on the advice and counsel of the community psychiatrist who clearly supported their decision to not force AL to attend a formal school program.

Recommendations Regarding Homebound Placement

Authors conclude that AL's homebound placement was inappropriate and non-therapeutic, and the prolonged acceptance of this educational placement by the school district raises questions about the adequacy of oversight for reliance on such restrictive measures.

As a general matter, rigorous scrutiny must be provided for students whose IEPs call for homebound status. The basis for such status must be regularly reviewed, with supporting documentation in the record, and with a rebuttable presumption that the child should eventually be transitioned to a less restrictive setting and a date set for return.

Attention must be paid to ensuring that all reasonable supports can be brought to bear to mitigate the reasons for the child's homebound placement, and no plan for homebound status should be approved by a district unless documentation is provided regarding such efforts. IEPs that approve homebound plans must also contain documentation that the planning team considered all relative benefits or consequences of such placement and why no alternatives were feasible.

Districts must be required to document for the State Department of Education, in real time, all students who are placed on homebound status, the basis for and expected duration of such status, the supports that were considered as an alternative to homebound placement, the supports that will be provided in accordance with the students' IEPS while the student is on homebound status, and when students will return to less restrictive settings. [61] Year-end data corresponding to such information should be included in reports to the State Department of Education.

The state/s may also want to consider an audit of existing homebound practices and procedures, and a needs assessment of the population of students who are currently or who have been placed on homebound within a certain timeframe. Based on this assessment, the state/s can determine how better to address practice concerns as well as target technical assistance or service development to support children with complex disabilities.

AGES 14 TO 18: HIGH SCHOOL

AL's developmental and mental health difficulties continued to become increasingly prominent as he entered high school, though many records indicate that he was able to function in the public high school environment, at least for a short time. According to Mr. Lanza, AL made an initial foray back into the public school system in 9th and 10th grade, but Mrs. Lanza later decided that keeping him home would be best. Mr. Lanza later stated that he saw AL as struggling with Obsessive Compulsive Disorder and Asperger's Syndrome, and that in some ways, it was a relief to have a diagnosis for him, and something the family could deal with and respond to. According to Mr. Lanza, AL saw his home as a comfort zone and felt that social interaction led to too much pressure. AL was not close with any of his relatives other than his older brother Ryan, though Mr. Lanza stated that by high school he and Ryan were not as close as they had been when they were younger.

Mr. Lanza described AL as very socially awkward at this time and spending an increasing amount of time with online gaming. AL enjoyed playing World of Warcraft on the computer and Mario Brothers on the gaming console. After Mr. Lanza moved to Stamford, he would try to have AL come and visit him, which AL would do sometimes. Eventually, however, AL stopped visiting with his father and after 2010 was not speaking with or communicating with his father at all.

Evaluation by Yale Child Study Center: October 24, 2006 (Ninth Grade)

In the fall of 2006, Mr. Lanza sought help through his Employee Assistance Program (EAP) to obtain a mental health referral for AL. At this point, AL's parents had been separated for five years. Per email correspondence from Mr. Lanza's EAP consultant, the family wanted to obtain "evaluation and treatment" for AL's Obsessive Compulsive Disorder. The family indicated, according to EAP coordinator, that the Lanzas would be willing to travel within the state "if there [was] a program/therapist to help their son, and them, as his disorder [was] significantly impacting the family as well." Mr. Lanza's emails indicate that the family was looking for a specialist who would be specifically knowledgeable about working with children diagnosed with Obsessive-Compulsive Disorder and Asperger's Syndrome.

---

[61] Currently states are required to report to the federal government the percentage of children with special education needs that are served in separate schools, residential facilities, or homebound/hospital placements.

On October 24, 2006, almost a year after the community psychiatrist first evaluated him, AL was seen at the Yale Child Study Center by a clinic psychiatrist. The evaluation was purportedly to determine if AL had Obsessive Compulsive Disorder in the context of a putative diagnosis of Asperger Syndrome.

It is not clear from the records why, if AL was already seeing a community psychiatrist, that Mr. Lanza sought additional help through his EAP. A later email by Mrs. Lanza to the *community* psychiatrist stated that Mr. Lanza thought it was "important" to get AL involved with the Yale Child Study Center and possibly get AL into a "teen support group over there." In present-day interviews, Mr. Lanza indicated that he had little direct involvement with the community psychiatrist and did not have any treatment records from that doctor.

Mrs. Lanza indicated at the time that she wanted the community psychiatrist's feedback on any recommendations possibly developed by the Yale Child Study Center because he had the "best understanding" of AL's situation. Mrs. Lanza acknowledged that Mr. Lanza was concerned over AL's socialization and that she had not really focused on that. She wrote that she had been "more concerned with keeping [AL] as comfortable as possible and just getting through each day."

The Yale psychiatrist's initial report observed that AL presented as a "pale, gaunt, and awkward young adolescent standing rigidly with downcast gaze and declining to shake hands."

AL's mother told the Yale psychiatrist that he used to look at people but did not anymore. AL then asked rhetorically, "Why should I have to." When the doctor explained all of the information that a person could learn by looking at a facial expression, such as a smile, AL stated that people could interpret smiles differently: "Some primates smile when they are frightened."

When asked for three magic wishes, AL could not think of any and instead he said that "he would wish that whatever was granting the wishes would not exist."

"Asked, 'What is a friend?' AL replied, 'It is difficult to define -- in whose culture do you refer?' Told 'AL's,' he replied, 'I do not know.' Asked whether he would like to have more friends, AL said no." According to the report, AL displayed a variety of rigid, controlling, and avoidant behaviors including his refusal to open doors for himself because he did not like to touch the doorknobs, and his worries about contamination of grease, dirt, and dust. AL was reported to be placing limits on his mother's behavior (e.g. by not allowing her to lean on things because it was improper). He had a variety of food rituals as well, related to texture. The doctor noted that AL had experienced a variety of marked changes in seventh grade, including no longer talking on the phone, using e-mail, or engaging in outdoor activities, and he had become increasingly socially withdrawn and reclusive. AL reportedly had not had any psychological testing.

The doctor noted that it was "difficult to interpret" AL's accelerated social withdrawal. However, the doctor considered that a "plausible explanation" might be that "social engagement (largely focused on activities) in the middle school years makes relatively few demands for social sophistication . . . . As [AL's] peers moved into early adolescence and middle school, the demands of social engagement changed dramatically, leaving AL feeling more inadequate or ostracized, setting off a cycle of withdrawal and avoidance."

The tone and level of urgency in the doctor's report appears a testament to his degree of concern. He references the use of medication to relieve symptoms, but is unclear whether AL would be willing to engage in efforts to reduce his anxiety and obsessive-compulsive behavior. The doctor's notes include the information that AL had been seen by the community psychiatrist for 10 visits and that he had urged anti-anxiety medication, which AL refused.

The psychiatrist stated that AL fell somewhere in the Pervasive Developmental Disorder or Autism Spectrum and he recommended further evaluation to clarify cognitive, social, and linguistic strengths and weakness. Psychological and speech and language evaluation was seen as essential. Treatment, the psychiatrist stated, would be difficult to implement outside of a broader therapeutic day school setting.

The psychiatrist then goes further, emphasizing his own words in italics:

> *Beyond the impact of OCD symptoms on himself and his mother, we are very concerned about AL's increasingly constricted social and educational world.* Much of emphasis has been on finding curricular level of instruction. Inability to tolerate even minimal interaction with even older more mature classmates will have grave consequences for his future education and social and occupational adaptation unless means of remediation are found. Inability to interact with classmates will prove increasingly deleterious to education. *We believe it is very important to reframe the discussion with school from issues of curricular content to much more urgent issues of how to accommodate AL's severe social disabilities in a way that would permit him to be around peers and to progress, rather than regress, socially, as well as academically.*

The psychiatrist went on to say,

> Understandably, AL's parents have gone to great lengths to compensate for AL's hypersensitivities and social difficulties and aversions by providing home-bound instruction.

> However we believe that there is a significant risk to AL in creating, even with the best of intentions, a prosthetic environment which spares him having to encounter other students or to work to overcome his social difficulties. Having the emphasis on adapting the world to AL, rather than helping him to adapt to the world, is a recipe for him to be a homebound recluse, unable to attend college or work productively into his twenties and thirties and beyond with mother becoming increasingly isolated and burdened.

The Yale psychiatrist wrote that AL clearly suffered from an impairing developmental disorder that qualified him for special education services. AL was unable to make effective use of social interactions with peers and social aversions precluded him from participating in classroom instruction. The psychiatrist indicated that it would be essential for the school to convene an IEP meeting to perform further psychological, speech, language, and occupational therapy assessments and develop an effective education plan. The psychiatrist further recommended that this process should include input from experts in Autism Spectrum/Pervasive Development Disorders.[62]

The Yale psychiatrist felt that AL required intensive help with social language use—using communication that is appropriate to setting, listener, context, or purpose. There was also a question as to whether AL could be helped with social disabilities and other developmental symptoms in a public high school or whether he needed a special therapeutic school setting tailored to bright children with developmental challenges. The psychiatrist appeared to consider such a therapeutic setting as optimal for addressing AL's "disabling OCD symptoms in the overall therapeutic context beyond what can be done piecemeal in weekly office-based therapy"—in part because behavioral, therapeutic approaches needed to be introduced in the context of AL's activities of daily living. Email correspondence between professionals at the clinic indicate that they felt AL needed "tons of special education support, with expert consultation," and underscored their view that he likely needed a therapeutic school setting.

Finally, the Yale psychiatrist noted that the family needed "tons of parental guidance—without that, any office based approach to his [challenges] will fail, certainly if it is without medication."

---

[62] "The diagnostic category of pervasive developmental disorders (PDD) refers to a group of disorders characterized by delays in the development of socialization and communication skills. Parents may note symptoms as early as infancy, although the typical age of onset is before 3 years of age. Symptoms may include problems with using and understanding language; difficulty relating to people, objects, and events; unusual play with toys and other objects; difficulty with changes in routine or familiar surroundings, and repetitive body movements or behavior patterns. Autism (a developmental brain disorder characterized by impaired social interaction and communication skills, and a limited range of activities and interests) is the most characteristic and best studied PDD. Other types of PDD include Asperger's Syndrome, Childhood Disintegrative Disorder, and Rett Syndrome. Children with PDD vary widely in abilities, intelligence, and behaviors. Some children do not speak at all, others speak in limited phrases or conversations, and some have relatively normal language development. Repetitive play skills and limited social skills are generally evident. Unusual responses to sensory information, such as loud noises and lights, are also common." *Pervasive Developmental Disorders*, NATIONAL INSTITUTE OF NEUROLOGICAL DISORDERS AND STROKE, http://www.ninds.nih.gov/disorders/pdd/pdd.htm (last visited Oct. 31, 2014).

Family Briefly Engages in Services with Yale

One day after AL's evaluation by Yale, Mrs. Lanza wrote an email to the doctor regarding the treatment recommendations. She indicated that AL would not agree to any sort of medication management as recommended. She wrote as follows:

> Thank you for taking the time to meet with AL yesterday . . . . I wanted to let you know that the options you presented are not going to work at this time. I would like to save you any further investment of your time.
>
> As I mentioned during the telephone conversation previous to our meeting, AL's OCD component is strongly tied to Asperger Syndrome and he is adamantly opposed to medication. The OCD component is now based on superstition or in an effort to influence outside events or luck. I thought I had been clear that I was looking for individual intervention, perhaps some sort of behavior modification, for the Asperger Syndrome foremost, sensory integration disorder, and the two OCD like components that are impacting his ability to attend school.
>
> His refusal to take medication would make it impossible for him to be part of the study group and will just further agitate him. He was quite angry about the line of questioning that the interview took. As you might expect from an Asperger child, he had no understanding of the metaphors, and was quite disturbed by the fairy godmother scenario you gave him. You mentioned that the wait list for treatment for Asperger is quite lengthy, and that the study group was the alternative. However, participation in a study group, with the implied possibility of medication, will not be helpful in this case. So while I very much appreciate your effort, this is not the right course of treatment for him.

The Yale psychiatrist responded quickly, acknowledging that given AL's reluctance to take medication (that the psychiatrist continued to believe was indicated), other options should be considered from the clinical research trial group. The Yale psychiatrist told Mrs. Lanza that the coordinator of the Pervasive Developmental Delay (PDD) group, an Advanced Practice Registered Nurse (APRN), was very knowledgeable about "treatment/education resources in the community," and that this individual would be happy to work with Mrs. Lanza and AL directly. Mrs. Lanza indicated that she would pursue working with that group and that she thought the doctor's report was "insightful" and many of his recommendations were "worth pursuing."

There was some indication that AL's mother did not think an Asperger's diagnosis really fit AL. She wrote in an email two days after the Yale evaluation that based on her research he did not "fit that mold." He did not, according to her, have a "preoccupation with one interest, the inability to carry on a two-sided conversation, [or] the absence of caring about other's expectations."[63]

---

[63] In fact, the Yale APRN that worked with AL after the initial evaluation also did not feel certain that AL had an Autism Spectrum Disorder, including Asperger's Syndrome. Rather, this clinician concluded that AL was primarily

She said that she felt "horrible" in the Yale interview process, and that AL was "frustrated, and angry and anxious" during the interview. "His palms were sweating so much that his shirt got wet and he looked like he could have cried at any moment." Mrs. Lanza said that she felt like he was "being tortured."

Mrs. Lanza wrote that the evaluation did not seem to have "even a glimmer of hope attached to it," and may have made things worse. She was concerned that AL was so angry about "the whole thing," that "short of strapping him down," she didn't think he would be willing to talk to another doctor for a long time.

Subsequent to the clinic's evaluation, AL was seen briefly by the APRN coordinator of the PDD group at the Yale Child Study Center. As described in an interview carried out by the Connecticut State Police, she had four face-to-face meetings with AL between October 2006 and February 2007. She also had a number of e-mail and telephone contacts with Mr. and Mrs. Lanza during that same time period. During the course of treatment (though not at the time of initial evaluation and meeting) the APRN became aware that AL was also being seen regularly by the *community* psychiatrist.[64] Both the Yale psychiatrist and APRN indicated during present-day interviews that they were not aware at the time evaluation and treatment started that AL was being concurrently seen by the community psychiatrist. Records reflect later conversations between the APRN and the community psychiatrist, but do not contain copies of any of that doctor's treatment records or evaluations.

AL was described by the APRN as "emotionally paralyzed" and severely limited in his ability to lead a normal life. During her conversations with him, he asked questions about schizophrenia and Obsessive Compulsive Disorder, but was unwilling to share if he was experiencing any of the symptoms of the disorders. She discussed with him the clinical components of these disorders and those of psychotic depression. She described AL as having "many rituals and prohibitions for his behavior and the behavior of others." AL agreed, in part, with the clinician that he was emotionally paralyzed by anxiety, but he did not feel that he suffered because of it, nor was he willing to take medication.

At one point, in February 2007, Mr. Lanza and the APRN discussed the trajectory of AL's treatment. Mr. Lanza indicated that AL did not want to continue going to Yale, that he was "angry" about having to attend and that he did not think the "process [would] help him." He also wanted his father present during sessions and did not think there was a benefit to meeting alone with the clinician. The APRN responded that she was in communication with AL's community psychiatrist and that their work was complementary and having some progress. The APRN indicated that the community psychiatrist also thought that she should "[s]tay involved for a while" so as to maximize treatment benefits for AL. With regard to AL's frustration with seeing the clinician, she stated:

---

debilitated by *anxiety* and Obsessive Compulsive Disorder. Whether these diagnoses were co-morbid with or, in lieu of an Autism Spectrum Disorder is unconfirmed.

[64] Not to be confused with the Yale Child Study psychiatrist.

The process of asking AL to talk with me directly about what is going on is critical. I appreciate that AL's view is that he wouldn't say anything differently if [the father] were in the room, but I think he's wrong. His judgment about how social/family dynamics work in a therapy situation is no more on target than his views regarding doorknobs and hand-washing . . . . He wants to control how the treatment goes because his anxiety is nearly unbearable if he can't feel he knows what's going to happen. I understand that. At the same time, he can't control the treatment because his thinking is distorted and irrational. I can't agree to follow his lead!

In fact, when I talk with him alone he has to respond, and last time I pushed him a bit. I am not surprised that he was angry, that's OK . . . . I told AL he has a biological disorder that can be helped with medication. I told him what the medicines are and why they can work.

I told him he's living in a box right now, and the box will only get smaller over time if doesn't get some treatment.

I'm fine to see him this week at 11. I am OK to talk with him and you at the beginning, but the session to address his issues has to be just him and me. I'd do it differently if I thought it would help, but I'm convinced it won't. Let me know your reactions.

Mr. Lanza responded that he would defer to the APRN's judgment in this matter.

Mrs. Lanza also sent the Yale report to the community psychiatrist looking for his feedback on the clinic's recommendations, and she asked if he would "take the lead role" in AL's treatment plan. The Yale APRN, after receiving permission from the Lanzas, also spoke with a Newtown school district professional regarding AL's presentation and treatment needs. Records do not indicate whether written materials were shared by Yale with the school, and the educational file *does not* contain a copy of the Yale psychiatrist's report.[65] Interviews indicate that there may have been differing expectations regarding the scope or extent of information-sharing between the school district and the Yale clinic. A copy of the school district's most recent psychological evaluation was shared with Yale and does appear in the Yale treatment records.[66]

In January, 2007, Mrs. Lanza wrote to the APRN to give her "feedback" on the most recent session.

"It was actually the best meeting AL has had with anyone. He was calm and conversational on the way home, which is very unusual.... As far as his comfort level ... it isn't just that he is painfully uncomfortable—he actually doesn't feel safe. He often tells me that he is frightened, even in our own

---

[65] A fax number for Newtown High School appears in the Yale record, indicating a need for the number to fax information from Yale to the school.

[66] The record does show an unrestricted, unlimited release signed by AL's parents permitting Yale to share all treatment information with Newtown Public Schools.

home and obviously more so in public. I think it is the fear that paralyzes him. His father will be bringing him over on Thursday so that I can get a couple of hours off, but please let me know if you need any input or if anything needs to be followed up at home."

Around February, 2007, Mr. Lanza wrote to the APRN that AL seemed to making progress. Mr. Lanza recounted a recent outing to the arcade and the mall with AL, where AL was able to visit a number of different stores. Mr. Lanza wrote that AL "ha[d] not wanted to do anything like that for over a year," and seemed to "enjoy the outing." Mr. Lanza wrote that "it appears the time that you are spending with AL may be paying off." Mr. Lanza said he would follow up with a new appointment date.

The feedback appeared to change after AL agreed, however reluctantly, to take the medication the APRN was prescribing. In late February, 2007 AL was prescribed a small dose of an anti-depressant/anti-anxiety medication by the APRN. Mr. Lanza strongly articulated his support of this direction in treatment. He told the APRN that despite AL's strong aversion, that he and Mrs. Lanza agreed that it was important for AL to try the medication. Mr. Lanza indicated that AL's judgment on medication was "no more appropriate than his judgment" on the value or logistics of therapy, and that these decisions should be left to the professionals and parents.

Mr. Lanza stated that he and Mrs. Lanza would sit down with AL and "explain" to him that they were "insist[ing]" he take the medication. According to Mr. Lanza, AL needed to understand that "as his parents [they] were responsible for his care and well-being and that in that capacity, [they] were] relying on the advice of a team of professionals" regarding treatment recommendations.

The APRN also spent time talking to AL about why he needed medication, and recommended a couple of books to him on Obsessive Compulsive Disorder. In later police interviews the APRN described AL's mother's response to her recommendations for medication as "non-compliant." Immediately after prescribing the medication, the clinician received a call from the mother reporting that AL was "unable to raise his arm." Mrs. Lanza stated that AL was attributing this symptom to the medication. An email from Mrs. Lanza to the clinic indicated that AL took the medication for three days. Mrs. Lanza wrote an email that AL experienced immediate and diverse symptoms associated with the medication, including "decreased appetitive and nausea . . . dizziness . . . disorientation," disjointed speech, and sweating. She stated that "he couldn't think. He sat in his room, doing nothing."

Despite the APRN's attempt to convince the mother that the medication could not be producing the problems with AL's arm, and that other symptoms could be managed with time and appropriate dosing, Mrs. Lanza said AL would be discontinuing the medication. The APRN urged Mrs. Lanza to encourage him to progress with the medication and noted that Mrs. Lanza observed a decrease in some of his obsessive-compulsive behaviors. Mrs. Lanza replied that AL's symptoms in response to the medication were very severe, that he was "practically vegetative," so he could not be seen as having improved. Mrs. Lanza stated, in an email, that she had consulted with the community psychiatrist regarding the side effects "and we decided to discontinue the meds," partly due to Mrs. Lanza's fear of side effects and partly to determine whether the side effects were "psychological."

Shortly after AL first took the prescribed medication in 2007, Mrs. Lanza reported to Mr. Lanza the strong side effects she observed. She wrote that the APRN was "wasting her time" with AL and that AL did not trust her, and that in fact he "loathed" her. She thought he would work better with the community psychiatrist as his primary support and that they should increase those visits in lieu of working with Yale. She wrote that AL had lost weight and couldn't "even pour his own cereal." Mr. Lanza appeared to agree with the new plan.

The family ultimately decided not to continue with the Yale Child Study Center. Mr. Lanza later stated in a present day interview that "AL was not open to therapy . . . . He did not want to talk about problems and didn't even admit he had Asperger's."[67] Records indicate that the parents agreed to see if the community psychiatrist could offer better help for AL. Again, the lack of documentation regarding AL's therapeutic relationship with the community psychiatrist hampers authors' ability to determine what different dynamics were involved there, what treatment was being provided, how goals were set, or how progress was being measured. Authors infer that the community psychiatrist may have facilitated more of an accommodation approach to AL.

In March, 2007, having not seen AL since the administration of medication, the Yale APRN contacted AL's community psychiatrist by email stating that all agreed it would be better for the family to "work with one provider," and that the "consensus" was that the community psychiatrist "would be the best person," given that AL really liked and trusted him.

Overall, the psychiatrist and APRN at Yale both indicated, in present-day interviews, their view that AL was profoundly impaired by anxiety and Obsessive Compulsive Disorder, and that his parents, and certainly AL, may not have understood the depth or implications of his disabilities. It may have been easier for the parents to accept that AL was a youth with a "high functioning" disorder, conceptualizing him as someone who was gifted but who had odd or challenging behaviors that needed behavioral modification.

The Yale APRN, in a present day interview, offered her view that AL may not, in fact, have had an Autism Spectrum Disorder, but rather that he suffered from disabling anxiety and Obsessive Compulsive Disorder. [68]

While it is not uncommon for parents to struggle to identify and accept their child as suffering a disabling impairment, the Yale Child Study Center clinicians who evaluated and treated AL felt that his parents, and certainly his mother, may have had greater than average difficulty with accepting the extent of AL's disabilities. Yale did not think that AL was gifted and unique, pointing to the average

---

[67] Solomon, *supra* note 34, at 13.
[68] Additional correspondence indicates that the Lanza family had some difficulty in obtaining reimbursement for evaluation and treatment services provided by Yale Child Study Center and that the Yale psychiatrist offered, in July 2007, assistance in obtaining such reimbursement from the insurer.

cognitive abilities captured by the school's psychological testing. Rather, Yale saw AL's singular appetites for certain types of learning as arising from his obsessive-compulsive tendencies, and that in actuality, he had average aptitude, and great deficits in certain areas. Yale saw Mrs. Lanza in particular as being controlled in some ways by AL, unwilling or unable to alter her style of coping and hyper-vigilant management of his symptoms. In some ways, Yale surmised that this constant placation of AL may have been why he did not feel that he suffered or was otherwise debilitated by his impairments. He did not need to suffer the weight of his problems, as his primary caretaker made every effort to keep him as comfortable as possible. Mrs. Lanza had great difficulty seeing the value in pushing AL out of this comfort zone. Her comment that she was "torturing" AL during his Yale evaluation echoes her earlier comment to a school administrator that she was "abusing" AL by keeping him in the Danbury Emergency Department.

Follow up to the Yale Child Study Recommendations

The Lanzas signed a release of information permitting exchange of any and all mental health and educational information about AL to be shared between the school district and the Yale Child Study Center. A treatment note indicates that the Lanzas wanted the APRN to provide her input to the school regarding AL's educational program. The APRN agreed to call the school to describe her understanding of AL's presentation. Documents and interviews indicate that a phone conversation took place between the APRN at Yale and a Newtown school psychologist. There is little documentation available about what information was specifically shared regarding AL or what recommendations were provided for educational planning. Records do not confirm whether the actual draft report[69] created by the Yale Child Study Center was shared pursuant to the release of information.[70]

Email correspondence from early 2007 demonstrates that Mr. Lanza repeatedly contacted school officials to coordinate information sharing between the district, the community psychiatrist and the Yale Child Study Center. Mr. Lanza wrote to the school that the "key" for AL succeeding in his educational goals would be for him to develop "the necessary coping skills," and that the mental health providers were "crucial in such a plan."

Mr. Lanza also inquired as to what family services were available pursuant to the IEP and whether those services would be developed separately or would be part of the IEP itself. Very significantly, Mr. Lanza inquired as to how the community psychiatrist and the Yale Child Study Center could be incorporated as part of the IEP team or as "related services" in AL's education plan—demonstrating a recognition that information-sharing and care coordination would be critical for AL to move forward.

---

[69] The Yale Child Study Center report, created by one of the Center's psychiatrists, remained in "draft" form and was never labeled "final."

[70] If obtained by the school district, the treatment records and recommendations should be in the educational file. OCA also spoke with or otherwise interviewed certain current and former school officials regarding this matter. Not all former administrators were available for interview.

The response from the school district confirmed that releases had been obtained and that school personnel would obtain the necessary information from the mental health providers and incorporate their recommendations into AL's education plan. Present-day interviews with school officials confirm that seeking such information, including written reports and recommendations from outside providers, would have been the standard practice. Mr. Lanza sent numerous emails to school personnel between January and March of 2007 to coordinate a planning meeting to discuss care coordination and the incorporation of related mental health services into AL's IEP. However, no meeting took place at this time.

A Newtown school psychologist's evaluation from December, 2006 noted that AL was seen by the Yale Child Study Center and that AL was diagnosed with Asperger's Syndrome, Obsessive Compulsive Disorder and sensory issues.[71] There is no indication in the school records, however, as to whether school personnel actually saw or considered Yale's recommendations for treatment and education planning. The IEP ultimately created by the school and family in 2007 did not reflect the recommendations contained in the Yale Child Study Center report.

In the spring of 2007 (9th grade), and after AL's January IEP meeting, Mr. Lanza investigated whether a private or specialized program may be available that would be appropriate for AL's needs. These efforts were made directly in response to the Yale Child Study's suggestion that AL might need a specialized school to meet his therapeutic and educational needs. At one point in May of 2007, Mr. Lanza also reached out to Stamford Public Schools to see what special education programming that district could provide if AL came to live with him.

The Lanzas (Mrs. Lanza was copied on most of the correspondence) did not ultimately identify a therapeutic program for AL, expressing some frustration with the difficult process. One private program for children with non-verbal learning disabilities and autism spectrum disorders responded to the Lanzas that AL's testing indicated his "need for a more therapeutic environment" than what the private school could provide. The program instead provided advice to the Lanzas that they work with an educational consultant that specialized in helping families meet the needs of children with nonverbal learning differences. Another program that purported to specialize in serving "bright" children who needed a non-traditional educational experience emphasized that it was "not a special education school," nor was it a school for children with emotional disturbance.

There is no documentation in the district's IEP records that consideration or recruitment of a therapeutic private program was considered or discussed by the team.

---

[71] Note that the Yale Child Study Center psychiatrist and APRN did not definitively determine that AL had Asperger's Syndrome. The Yale psychiatrist opined, at the time of the evaluation that AL *may* fall on the Autism Spectrum.

Ongoing relationship with the community psychiatrist

Despite the lack of available treatment records and the community psychiatrist's present-day statements to interviewers that his tenure with AL was relatively brief, records indicate ongoing payment by the Lanzas to this psychiatrist for at least two years (through 2007), with one payment in 2008. There is no documentation in the pediatric or educational record of what treatment was being provided at this time or what input this doctor may have had for educational planning, or whether input would have been provided to Mrs. Lanza or to the school directly. School records contain no documentation of input from the community psychiatrist past early 2006 and no copies of any treatment recommendations. School records also contain no documentation of phone correspondence between school personnel and this psychiatrist.[72] Mrs. Lanza stated that she would be providing a particular staff member with the psychiatrist's phone number. School records contain no documentation from early 2006 forward of ongoing input regarding mental health issues.

Accordingly, while AL did have multiple IEP planning meetings with the school, there is no documentation that he received the special education supports and "expert consultation" so strongly recommended by the Yale Child Study Center. Despite Mr. Lanza's documented efforts to ensure careful care coordination between providers, these recommendations were either not obtained or were not integrated into the education plan.

Educational Review: High School

AL Returned to Public School in 9th Grade

As AL approached the 9th grade, his parents and the school agreed to ease him back into a school environment. The school would move in very small steps, first re-introducing him to school personnel through personal contacts and individual tutoring. A former special education administrator for Newtown Public Schools remembers during her one conversation with AL's community psychiatrist (possibly during AL's 8th grade year), that the doctor predicted they would *never* get AL back in school because he was the "most anxious" youth the doctor had ever seen.
In November of the 9th grade (2006), the IEP team recommended a psychological evaluation for AL—to be conducted by the school district—and the parents agreed. At this time AL had been receiving tutoring for major academic subjects (up to 10 hours) but had also begun to come to the High School for a combination of tutoring and classroom work in Chemistry, Math, and Latin, depending on his ability to handle the environment.

The community psychiatrist's previous description, recommendations, and diagnosis of Asperger's Disorder were still noted in the educational record, and the notes regarding AL's "present

---

[72] At least one email authored by Mrs. Lanza in February, 2007 indicates that she was connecting school personnel with the community psychiatrist so that he could provide input on modifying AL's history curriculum. Another email from Mrs. Lanza to the community psychiatrist indicates that school personnel wanted the psychiatrist to connect directly with a district psychologist regarding recommended changes to AL's curriculum and that the school was open to any curricular changes or other ideas, including "independent study."

performance" levels reflected that his high level of anxiety, Asperger's characteristics, Obsessive-Compulsive disorder, and sensory issues were impacting his performance to a significant degree.

The district's psychological testing indicated that AL's ability to sustain attention, concentrate, and exert mental control were in the superior range. AL also displayed a strong ability to attend to and hold information in short-term memory while performing some operation or manipulation with the information. AL demonstrated exceptional auditory working memory and attention skills. However, he would be expected to struggle slightly with comprehending novel information. His relatively low score on the Comprehension subtest included responses to each item but not always with a "socially sensitive" response. There was no discussion of the qualitative nature of these responses.

Overall, while some of AL's academic skills were assessed to be in the very superior range, his cognitive abilities tested as "average' and he had difficulty with stimuli that involved faces or objects related to social experiences.[73]

The district's psychological evaluation concluded that there was no evidence of a specific learning disability, and that school issues were primarily related to AL's identified emotional and/or Pervasive Developmental Disorder behaviors. It was recommended that AL continue to be eased into regular classroom time as his comfort level increases and anxiety decreases. Desensitization was referenced, with recommendations for small classes, *but without any direct therapeutic support.*

The IEP team meeting held in January of AL's 9th grade year (2007), ostensibly to review the district's psychological evaluation and develop an Individualized Education plan, provides no evidence that the evaluation findings were discussed. There was no assessment of social-emotional behavior, despite its having been cited in the record as the reason for AL's homebound placement. This IEP team classified AL as eligible for special education with a primary disability of Other Health Impairment[74] (rather than the more apt eligibility categories of Autism or Emotional Disturbance) and the IEP team created an education plan almost entirely without reference to AL's social-emotional difficulties, except to say that his anxiety disorder, Asperger Syndrome, compulsive disorder, and rigidity impacted his learning in a regular education environment as well as his ability to take part in a general education curriculum.

AL's difficulty in communicating with others was also identified as impacting his ability to participate in a regular education environment. However, the only goal to address these crippling and multiple

---

[73] The district's psychological evaluation incorporated the use of standardized tools such as the Woodcock Johnson and the WISC-IV.

[74] OHI is an enumerated disability in special education law that means the student has "limited strength, vitality or alertness including a heightened alertness to environmental stimuli, that results in limited alertness with respect to the educational environment, that

    1.   is due to chronic or acute health problems such as asthma, attention deficit disorder or attention deficient hyperactivity disorder, diabetes, epilepsy, or heart condition, hemophilia, lead poisoning, leukemia, nephritis, rheumatic fever, and sickle cell anemia; and Tourette Syndrome, and

    2.   adversely affects a student's educational performance."

34 C.F.R. § 300.8(c)(9) (2013). OHI was not the appropriate classification, however, for AL, who should have been classified as having either Autism or Emotional Disturbance.

disabilities was to "increase time with others in a school setting." No performance criteria or evaluative procedures were included beyond teacher observation. There were no speech and language related services in the IEP.

The required consideration of special factors—"For students whose behavior impedes his or her learning or that of others, the PPT [Term for IEP team used in Connecticut] has considered strategies, including positive behavioral interventions and supports to address that behavior"—received a response of "Not Applicable." Again a single statement addresses his ongoing removal from the regular education environment "because AL requires more intensive service than provided for in a regular education classroom at this time." However, the services offered were essentially 10 hours of academic tutoring.

It appears from available email correspondence and treatment notes from the Yale Child Study Center that communication between the district psychologist and Yale did take place *after* the January IEP meeting.

Both Mr. and Mrs. Lanza were present at the next IEP meeting in May 2007. There continued to be no evaluation of social-emotional behavior, although the IEP "requires removal of the student from the regular education environment because AL requires more intensive service than provided for in a general education classroom." The location of services was simply described as "in-district." No accommodations or modifications were described, except for use of a laptop. There was no information in the record regarding AL's current levels of performance, strengths, needs or the impact of the disability. There were no targeted objectives with specific criteria.

Despite the telephone call between the Yale Child Study Center and the school psychologist, there is no reference to the Yale recommendations in the IEP. There is no reference to the Yale psychiatrist's recommendation for additional communication and occupational therapy evaluations, or for the inclusion of input from an expert in the education of children with Autism Spectrum and Pervasive Developmental Disorders.

However, present-day interviews and correspondence from 2007 indicate that all involved felt AL was making progress. School staff and family were somewhat successful in getting AL to leave his house and at least enter the school building. He was able to work one-on-one with teachers and was beginning to tolerate the presence of other adults and students. As the school year progressed, district staff attempted to try AL in some small groups and have him work, at times, in a less isolated fashion. While AL was not working directly with a skilled behaviorist, therapist or other professional with expertise in educating children with developmental or mental health disorders, the district and family were having some success de-sensitizing AL to the school environment.

An unsigned report from May 2007 (spring of AL's 9th grade year) also confirms that AL made some progress during the 9th grade year. He was scheduled to have a speech evaluation and take a computer class. However, by June, AL had been seen for medical treatment because of irritated hands related to obsessive compulsive hand washing. The note (possibly from the school nurse) stated that he continued to be followed without medications by the community psychiatrist and that a referral had been made to another doctor for a neurology workup.[75] There is no ongoing correspondence beyond 2006, or any exchange of treatment records between the community psychiatrist, a neurologist, and the district. It does not appear that the speech and language evaluation ever took place.

"Student wants to return to school as a typical high school student."

The educational team began to prepare to mainstream AL for 10th grade (2007-08 school year), moving him from reliance on one-to-one tutoring to participation in classes. A note from the school nurse in August 2007 appeared to be preparing school personnel for AL's return to the high school in the fall and noted that his goal was to be a typical student.

In the nurse's note AL was described as presenting with "high functioning" Asperger's Syndrome and anxiety.[76] He was described by the nurse as "bright" and not wanting to be "defective." The nurse stated that he wanted to be in school to increase his knowledge. AL was described in this note as having come a "long way" with his "crisis team" and assistance from a trusted school employee: the head of security.

These records appear to reflect an ongoing underestimation of AL's actual disabilities. Although AL's putative diagnosis from the community psychiatrist was Asperger's Syndrome (also noted in the pediatric medical record), the Yale Child Study Center clinicians did not conclude that AL was "high functioning" or that he definitively had Asperger's Syndrome. Rather, they saw him as profoundly impaired and debilitated by anxiety, with extensive special-education/therapeutic needs. In actuality, there was some overlap in diagnostic and descriptive language between practitioners, as the community psychiatrist appeared to agree with Yale that AL was grossly and primarily debilitated by anxiety, describing AL to one school official as "the most anxious [youth] he had ever seen."

The nurse noted a list of preparations for AL to come to class early, leave later from the classroom, and his continuing high level of anxiety, germ phobia, and sensitivity to smells. The note emphasized that communications with AL must be very clear:

> It is 'more scary if he does not understand and rocks and withdraws. Being unclear can be devastating to this child and his family.' He was to be brought to the nurse [if injured?] because he cannot process pain. He is non-emotional. He was to e-mail teachers if he wanted to ask questions. There was concern that fire drills 'might freak him out.' This was to be addressed by having a teacher stay with him.

Several days later, on August 26, 2007 (pre-10th grade), a communication from a psychiatrist stated that the doctor had reviewed AL's history with Mrs. Lanza and that he was confident that AL was prepared and ready to attend Newtown High School as a full time student that fall. Authors spoke

---

[75]AL's available medical records, including his pediatric records, do not confirm that a neurology evaluation ever took place.

to this doctor, whose name does not appear elsewhere in the medical record, and confirmed that the doctor was covering for AL's treating psychiatrist in the community. This doctor may have written the letter strictly on the basis of communications from AL's mother.[77]

During the scheduled PPT on August 27, 2007, AL's mother raised a new fear that AL would not report difficulties he encountered during the school day. She said that his sensory-motor integration deficit might prevent him from realizing that he had been injured. It is unclear whether this was an indirect concern about bullying or simply a new, previously unstated, concern.

Mrs. Lanza also stated that AL really wanted to return to school. She wrote to a school staff member before school began that he "insists on walking through that front door," and that he was "prepared." The PPT and resulting Education Plan still listed AL's special education classification as Other Health Impaired and articulated the plan for him to return full time to school. The classification in the education record of Other Health Impaired is concerning, since OHI is not the appropriate classification for a youth with significant developmental and mental health challenges.

Rather, "OHI, per . . .," is a classification designed for students with limited strength, vitality or alertness, including a heightened alertness to environmental stimuli, that results in limited alertness with respect to the educational environment due to chronic or acute health problems such as asthma, attention deficit disorder or attention deficit hyperactivity disorder, diabetes, epilepsy, a heart condition, hemophilia, lead poisoning, leukemia, nephritis, rheumatic fever, and sickle cell anemia; and adversely affects a child's educational performance.[78]

By this point, there were multiple indicators that AL met statutory-regulatory criteria and applicable guidance for *autism spectrum disorders* or, alternatively, for *emotional disturbance*. These classifications on his educational record would have more aptly identified his challenges and created different expectations for his plan, such as what disciplines were needed for appropriate educational planning and what types of goals, objectives and services (addressing communication, peer relationships and therapeutic goals) should be included in his Individual Education Plan. In fact, the Connecticut State Department of Education had published a comprehensive guide for districts, dated 2005, outlining best practices regarding the identification, evaluation and educational planning for children on the autism spectrum.[79] Adherence to this guidance would have fostered much greater focus on behavior, communication, social-emotional health, and adaptive skills.

---

[77] Per present day efforts by authors to obtain AL's medical records, correspondence from a healthcare provider indicated that the doctor who authored the above-referenced note may have "taken over" patients from the community psychiatrist that had previously seen AL.

[78] 34 C.F.R § 300.7(c)(9) (2013).

[79] Connecticut State Department of Education, *Guidelines for Identification and Education of Children and Youth with Autism*, (2005) http://www.sde.ct.gov/sde/cwp/view.asp?a=2626&q=322672

Another relevant guide from the State Department of Education also existed (dated 1997) for the assessment and provision of services to children with Emotional Disturbance.[80] This comprehensive technical assistance manual specifically reminds districts of their obligations to evaluate (or ensure and obtain evaluation information regarding) youth suspected of having a mental health disorder in all relevant domains: psychological, medical, developmental, and social. Districts are advised to incorporate into the IEP information about the social and personal competencies needed to maximize students' independence. The guide even included checklists to ensure creation and documentation of IEP program components in all areas relevant to the student's needs:

- Education in the least restrictive environment
- Individual Transition Planning
- School-based counseling [if needed]
- Consultation
- Behavior management
- Family collaboration
- Crisis Plan
- Performance Monitoring and data collection.[81]

By not classifying his needs appropriately, attention to AL's severe disabilities focused, as the Yale psychiatrist previously warned, on *curricular issues* rather than on the social and emotional characteristics that were seriously impacting his ability to participate in a regular educational environment.

The absence of a plan to address AL's social-emotional issues with a program that was sufficiently intense and therapeutic likely contributed to a situation in which he eventually became increasingly withdrawn and socially isolated. Yet, despite ample evidence to suggest that AL's disability would prevent his success in a mainstream high school setting, the IEP states: "[s]tudent will participate fully in regular classes."

Despite the lack of appropriate and expert-driven educational programming, school staff and Mrs. Lanza were well engaged with each other and making many efforts to accommodate and facilitate AL's attendance in school. School staff communicated regularly with Mrs. Lanza regarding AL, with many communications indicative of investment and interest in AL's success. Mrs. Lanza also maintained a *very* close eye on AL's programming and curriculum. She engaged in a series of communications with teachers at the high school concerning the details of AL's day.

She informed one of AL's teachers that he worried about dying, being bullied, and that he was acutely aware that he was different from other kids. She feared that any story that referenced these social issues in a way that AL could identify with would bring on periods of insomnia and a loss of appetite.

---

[80] Connecticut State Department of Education, *Guidelines for Identification and Education of Children and Youth with Serious Emotional Disturbance (1997).*
[81] *Id.* at 28 – 30.

Mrs. Lanza also noted, "[a]nother thing we might have trouble with is boy-meets-girl type [of literature]. An adapted reading list is being provided as a substitute for the standard curriculum." In another note, Mrs. Lanza states:

> AL has indicated that he would like to try to learn about symbolism and use of figures of speech. Can you suggest any good books on the subject?

A series of emails between Mrs. Lanza and school personnel concerning AL's program follows. He was originally scheduled (8/27/07) to take Sociology, AP U.S. History, AP Chemistry, AP Physics, English, Math, and Latin—a plan which did not last beyond a few months.

AL also joined the Technology Club at the start of 10th grade and his participation in this student group was a notably positive development. Records indicate that AL developed a good relationship with the club's faculty advisor and that he was able, during this time period, to mix with the other students in the club and participate in club activities. Certainly at this point, progress had indeed been made since the time when AL would not leave his house and attend school at all. Efforts to de-sensitize AL to his environment and manage his experience in the high school were having some positive effect and may have obfuscated the ongoing need for mental health support and consultation with the educational team.

Mrs. Lanza expressed written appreciation for the work of the school team with AL. She stated that she was "impressed" with one particular school staff who helped him return to regular classes at the high school, even when Mrs. Lanza thought they had run into a "brick wall." Mrs. Lanza commended this individual as having had "tenacity and creativity to find the doorways in that wall." Mrs. Lanza described a group of teachers and counselors who were assigned to work with him, and that as a "parent of a child with special needs," she appreciated the group leader's "accessibility, positive attitude, and [ ] ability to handle any situation that [arose]."

Emails exchanged between Mrs. Lanza and school personnel also repeat Mrs. Lanza's observation that AL did not want to be identified as a special education student and that he did not want special accommodations. In one email, Mrs. Lanza states that he did want to be in school regularly but that he equated a "small classroom setting" to being a "[s]tupid class." Repeatedly, however, Mrs. Lanza's emails note that he struggled tolerating other students, their presence or behavior, in certain classes. According to Mrs. Lanza, AL wanted more "independent study." Mrs. Lanza apologized to school staff via email and stated that she knew he was "a difficult case, and [that] everyone [was] working very hard to accommodate [him]." She stated that she just wanted to make his "experience at school as tolerable as possible."

Given the lack of therapeutic supports provided to AL, it is noteworthy that many emails going back and forth document his challenges, anxieties, and difficulties being in class. A staff member from the school wrote in 2007 that they were "optimistic for AL because there are so many good people who will support him" and that staff should "not hesitate" to contact Mrs. Lanza because she had "done an amazing job under very difficult circumstances and [would] be willing to do anything [she could] to help AL be successful."

Mr. Lanza was very supportive of AL's academic pursuits, and there are multiple emails between them as AL sought advice or information regarding class schedule or even career opportunities in the sciences.

Emails show that school personnel appeared vested in seeing him succeed. One undated email exchange depicted one school staff stating:

> OH MY GOSH! AL is ready to join my class??? I HAD BETTER GET READY! I'm so nervous! Let's talk . . . are they starting with a short visit or two or jumping right in and seeing how it goes with the potential to leave early as needed??? What about "prepping" my class before his arrival --- today I have an appointment at 2:30 . . . but we can talk on the phone tonight . . . .

The response from the coordinator is indicative of the school district's approach to AL:

> My guess is that he will start with an entire class. In my past experience, observing a class is more difficult than participating in a class. As for your other students—when in doubt – IGNORE AL. Any attention is tough. In terms of prepping them – just think about what you know about AL.
>
> - No loud noises
> - No strong smells
> - No sudden movements
> - No unpredictable actions, noises, smells, etc.
> - Speak with a purpose or "Let me work."
> - AL may be uncomfortable around the boys, but I don't know that for sure.
>
> I am sure he will tell us whatever is a problem . . . . .
>
> Have you talked to [STAFF MEMBER] about the math he needs for your class? Would you like me to do that? So many questions! At least our jobs are never dull.

There are times when emails between Mrs. Lanza and school staff were being exchanged every day of the week. The tone of the emails—which were often efforts to specifically manage AL's day or his academic experience—was often one of cordiality and even partnership.

It is clear in the correspondence as well from present-day interviews with district personnel, that the educational team felt they were "thinking outside the box" for AL, and making deliberate and well-intended efforts to meet AL's complex needs through careful and extensive partnership with his mother. However, the emails appear indicative of a partnership around a strategy of habituation, or even of appeasement, without a skilled, therapeutic, expert-driven approach that would help AL adapt to the world. One email from Mrs. Lanza reflects the lengths the educational team went to adapt the world to AL rather than help AL adapt to the world:

> "He will not accept any preferential treatment at all. Since he obviously NEEDS preferential treatment, it leaves me scurrying around behind his back fixing things… i.e. The gym thing. I actually had to make up a story about liability, bureaucracy, and being out of school for over 12 months, etc. … then I have to go to [school staff] and get her to back that up … then I have to go to [another school staff], and get him to go along. Then his … teacher slips up and tells him that his IEP allows him to get out of study halls and I have to get her to recant and say it was a misunderstanding on her part. This is a high stress, 24/7 operation of misinformation. He does NOT have to go to lunch, but obviously I have to come up with a story that he will buy and then get everyone on the same page. Thanks for giving me the heads up… [about lunch]. I will get on it first thing in the morning. I will think of something. He wants to believe that he is an ordinary student, and I think it is important to let him believe for his self-esteem."

As the Yale Child Study Center noted in its previous evaluation of AL, management of AL's symptoms would not be enough to help him and would ultimately thwart his progress. He needed intense therapeutic and behavioral supports, responsive to his psychiatric disabilities, so that he could meaningfully build skills and sustain progress.

By February of that school year AL had dropped most of his mainstream classes, including Sociology, History, Chemistry, and Physics and had arranged to complete English as an "independent study." These decisions were communicated through Mrs. Lanza's contact with the school. It became clear that the recommendation for full time participation in regular classes was a goal that could not be met at that time.

At this point, there is no record of assistance in educational planning from the community psychiatrist who had seen AL through 2006, and little or no involvement from clinical professionals available to the school district, whether a school social worker, occupational therapist, behaviorist, or staff/consulting psychiatrist.

In March, Mrs. Lanza was again contemplating home-schooling AL, but worried that he would later be unable to show (a college?) all of his work with the Technology Club or work study. Summer of 2008 records indicate that AL was to receive Extended School Year Services (ESY), in the form of one-on-one tutoring from school staff. ESY services are for youth who, due to the nature of their disabilities, need an extended school year to continue to make progress with their educational goals.[82] Services may include academic and related services, such as speech and language support, occupational therapy, therapeutic supports, or any other appropriate interventions, individualized to the needs of the particular student.

---

[82] 34 C.F.R § 300.106 (2013).

In the fall of 2008, AL entered 11th grade and records indicate that he was still enrolled in the public high school. His IEP continued to classify him as Other Health Impaired and continued to offer him 10 hours of tutoring a week and a shortened school day, pending doctor's approval. AL did not re-enter mainstream classes in the high school again.

AL communicated his goal of graduating early from high school, and staff worked with him to assist with earning the necessary credits. By the beginning of AL's junior year, he had accumulated 11.5 credits towards the required 20 for graduation. By the end of the year, he was credited with 21, which allowed him to graduate a year early and exit special education services.

The 11th grade Individualized Education Plan also explicitly states that the team was recommending an updated release of information to speak with AL's community psychiatrist and that the district would contact the psychiatrist for an updated needs assessment. Records indicate that AL may not have been seen by the psychiatrist in many months. There is no documentation as to whether district personnel followed up on the stated recommendations in the IEP to connect with the psychiatrist or whether they tried and failed to obtain updated treatment records. If AL was no longer seeing a mental health professional in the community, the district should likely have determined that fact.

Mrs. Lanza reported that AL was taking classes at Western Connecticut State University during the 11th grade year as part of his "independent study." His GPA was reported as 3.89. The school team agreed to consider granting high school credit for college assignments but did not support funding the family's unilateral decision to enroll AL in college. A curriculum was cobbled together with Mrs. Lanza playing a role in selecting the books AL would read. She continued to report that his ability to attend high school was negatively and significantly impacted by his acute anxiety and asserted that he functioned better when his class work was concentrated into a single time block as in a college setting. Mr. Lanza communicated regularly with AL regarding potential course work and college classes. He also connected with a consultant on college education for youth with Autism Spectrum disorders to gain insight and advice to help prepare AL for post-secondary experience.

There remained no goals and objectives in the IEP addressing his social and emotional needs. The IEP did state as "goals" that AL would advocate for his personal and academic needs in tutoring sessions and the IEP noted that college courses were approved for high school credit each semester.

The IEP indicates that no other options to the tutoring and shortened day were considered. His transition plan stated only that he would enroll in classes that prepare for post-secondary education. Federal and state law require that special education plans include detailed and individualized transition goals and objectives for youth to help them successfully skill build and prepare for post-secondary experience. These transition plans should include attention to academic, social-emotional, and independent living skills. Transition support services can be provided even after a disabled youth has acquired all high school academic credits. Services must be individualized to the needs of the individual student, and include therapeutic, academic and functional daily living supports. Repeatedly, AL's transition plans as written in his IEPs were sparsely written and did not reflect the needs presented by his profound disabilities.

However, interviews with school staff indicate that despite the paucity of documentation, there was some attention to AL's transition needs. Efforts were made to connect AL, through a job coach, with an employer in the community. AL interned with and was later employed for a time by an individual in the community for whom AL did computer work. A written letter from this employer dated March 2009 indicated that AL was working "as an independent contractor" to resolve computer problems. The author of the letter indicated that AL was "cordial, professional" and displayed "expert attributes."

Members of AL's educational team stated in present-day interviews that they felt the district met AL's needs as they presented at the time. They felt that AL made definitive progress towards graduation readiness. He was able to return to the high school, at least for a time, and he was able to attend classes for some time. He participated in a student group, and he obtained some job skills and experience in the community, which his team *believed* demonstrated career readiness. His goal of graduating early and attending college classes did not seem inappropriate for a youth the school saw as "gifted," (despite information to the contrary in the school psychologist's report) with a voracious appetite for learning.

However, it is not clear how the IEP team members responded to AL's relatively short-lived participation in mainstream classes or a peer group. By 11th grade he was not able or willing to attend high school with his peers and there was nothing in his IEP that reflected consultation with a mental health professional, behaviorist, or any other individual experienced in educating youth with significant developmental or mental health needs. Notably, AL's IEP consistently stated that his transition skills, including his "daily living skills" were "age appropriate," while simultaneously noting his significant mental health disabilities.

The annual review of AL's IEP for the 2008–09 school year continued goals from the previous education plan and noted that he would, in fact graduate early and therefore exit special education services on June 26, 2009. Email correspondence between Mr. and Mrs. Lanza indicates that, at least at times, AL continued to struggle with aspects of his educational plan:

> June, 2009: "He wouldn't go to the tutor today. He seemed like he would all along … I checked with him several times during the day and he said he would go, and even 10 minutes before we should leave he was getting ready to go, but then had a meltdown and began to cry and couldn't go. He said things like its pointless, and he doesn't even know what he doesn't know. I tried everything to assure him and let him know it wouldn't matter if he hadn't finished the work, or couldn't finish, or didn't understand, and that's what the tutor would figure out … even if we go back and review Algebra 1 … but he couldn't stop crying, so I said we could try again next week."

> July, 2009: "Something must have gone wrong with class today. He wouldn't speak on the way home and had his hood completely covering his face. He went straight to his room and won't eat. I gave him time alone to compose and have tried to speak to him twice now, but he just keeps saying "It does

not matter" and "leave me" "I don't want to speak of it." Did you look at the syllabus? Is it possible he has already missed a deadline or not been prepared for a quiz/test? I don't know what I should do. I don't want to try to talk to him again because he sounds like he is on the verge of crying."

Correspondence between the special education teacher and the guidance counselor noted that he did not wish to participate in any graduation activities but that he would like to receive his diploma and a handshake from the principal.

It is important to note that youth with disabilities who receive special education services are eligible for academic and transition services through *age 21* if the continued provision of services is necessary to assist with making educational progress and in achieving agreed-upon goals and objectives. In fact, a youth may complete all academic requirements for graduation but continue with transition services for a year or even more, working on independent living skills and other goals necessary for transition to post-secondary life.[83] Here, AL not only had a paucity of transition planning, he graduated *early* from high school.

Medical Records 2006–2009

In June 2006, the medical record again documents AL's raw hands due to over-washing. This note echoed a medical record from 2003 documenting his excoriated skin due to hand washing. The 2006 record indicates AL was again prescribed Aquaphor. There is no documented follow up or coordination between the pediatrician and the community psychiatrist that he was purportedly seeing at that time.

A note from June 2006 indicates that Mrs. Lanza wanted to set up a consultation to discuss AL's weight loss. An August 2006 visit confirms weight and health concerns, and trouble sleeping. AL was 94 pounds at that time. The record indicated that he was "home schooled."[84]

The August 2006 note also states that he was referred to a pediatric neurologist, though there is no record that a neurology evaluation took place. And there is no letter or report in the pediatric record from any consulting neurologist, or even from the community psychiatrist that was referenced in the pediatric records from this time.

The September 2006 well-child record documents that AL was diagnosed with Obsessive Compulsive Disorder, Anxiety and Asperger's Syndrome, and that he was to seek or was seeking psychiatric care in the community.

There is sparse mention in his pediatric medical records of a discussion or plan for the mental health issues that he was exhibiting or was otherwise noted to have. There is no copy in the pediatric record

---

34 C.F.R § 300.106 (2013).

of the report and recommendations from Yale Child Study Center. The records, in fact, do not mention or reference this evaluation in any way.

AL's record indicates that he was seen for a variety of physical complaints over the years (chest pain, extremity pain, ear pain, eye pain, and repeat sore throat). Mrs. Lanza, who it seems was the parent who typically took AL to the doctor, did not check off that he had any mental health issues on an adolescent questionnaire contained in the medical record.

The February 2008 note states that AL continued to be diagnosed with Asperger's and Obsessive Compulsive Disorder but did not indicate what, if any, treatment was being provided or should be provided. In fact the well-visit form indicates that despite these issues, AL was receiving "no meds, and no psych." Under the heading "Development," next to sub-headings for "school," "after school activities," and "peer relations," nothing is written except "10th grade." The record notes that he was 112 pounds and almost 5 feet, 10 inches tall, suggesting possible anorexia at this time.

A subsequent note in the medical record, dated August 2008, indicated that he had a history of constipation (possibly linked to his weight and nutrition issues) and was prescribed Miralax to symptomatically respond to this concern.

There was no documentation of any counseling or referral regarding AL's weight, repetitive behaviors or other mental health issues after the 2006 note that he was following up with a community psychiatrist. No record indicates there were any significant school problems, though the records occasionally note that he was "home schooled" or on "independent study." His educational status could have been a major red flag of unaddressed developmental or mental health needs. A record from March 2009 indicates that school was going "much better," and that there continued to be no psychiatric involvement.

A 2009 medical record also indicates that AL was 5 feet, 10 inches tall and still weighed only 112 pounds. The same adolescent well-visit form indicates that the provider checked off that "anticipatory guidance" was provided regarding all issue areas contained on the form, including "nutrition advice," "siblings/peer relationship" and "internet safety." On the same form, under the heading "Development," the provider noted that AL was in 11th grade and attending community college. Under "concerns," it was noted that he had Asperger's Syndrome and Obsessive Compulsive Disorder. Nothing was written under "after school activities" or "peer relations." Under "Assessment," the provider checked off "well child/normal growth and development."

AL's Experiences with Other Youth in High School

During law enforcement/investigative interviews, several individuals who knew or interacted with AL discussed their impressions of him during high school. In 2007 and 2008, (AL's 10th grade) he belonged to the high school technology club and appeared to socially mix, to some degree, with the other students.

Multiple teachers and students attested, during interviews by the State Police, that they had been unaware of bullying or teasing incidents that might have negatively affected AL socially and emotionally. In fact, most who had known him during his school years described him as quiet, bright, reluctant to participate, and somewhat odd in that he carried a briefcase rather than a backpack and wore clothes that were too big. One former student referenced his tendency to pull his sleeves down over his hands if he was required to touch objects in the course of a class.

Whether bullying was an actual part of the picture of social isolation is unclear, but a history of bullying incidents is not supported by available documents. Still, most bullying occurs out of sight of staff and may be ignored or tolerated by the peer group. Furthermore, children with autism are known for not reporting even severe bullying because of poor self-advocacy and self-observation skills. Here, some youth later stated that they did not remember bullying but thought it would not be surprising if bullying had occurred. Accordingly, while the authors cannot completely confirm that bullying did not occur, there is no evidence that it did.

One youth from Technology Club later described AL in present day interviews as "a quiet kid . . . somewhat anxious because of facial expressions and an upright posture when he walked . . . the only odd behavior [that AL had] was pulling his sleeves over his hands any time he was handed an object from someone. AL wiped [the object] down with his sleeves before he would touch it." The same individual reported that though AL was "quiet," he was also sociable as long as he was included in conversation. However, the individual stated that AL would not "initiate" social conversation.

Another individual who had also participated in Technology Club with AL described "Local Area Network" computer parties that the children hosted or participated in during high school. This individual indicated that he had attended a LAN party at AL's house in 2008. Youth would bring laptops and play games online. When AL hosted the LAN party, nothing unusual happened, and he asked other students to take off their shoes and be "respectful of the house." This individual stated that "the only odd things that he remembers about AL was that he would sometimes not talk even if you were speaking directly to him, and that he wore the same shirt repeatedly." This individual stated that he did not remember AL talking about violence or any violent things.

AL was described as quiet, but also very smart. "When a question came up [AL] always had an answer." He was described as very smart in math, he "typically had a pocket protractor, calculator, almost a stereotype of high school nerd." AL was described as wearing a "green plaid button down short sleeved shirt over and over." One individual observed that while AL participated in the Technology Club activities and parties, it wasn't clear if he "had real friends to hang out with." One youth stated that no one appeared to "pick on" AL, that he tended to keep to himself, and "no one had a problem with him at all." He was described by one individual as "the smartest kid in tech club."

Another former student who was a year ahead of AL in school talked about his experiences with AL in the Technology Club. At one time, he lived close to AL's house in the Lanza's neighborhood and they rode the same school bus. This individual would sometimes ride next to AL on the bus. Like other youth, this individual also stated that AL would sometimes talk, but that he was "mostly quiet and kept to himself." He "dressed nicely, tucked in button down shirt, pocket protector with pens." The individual did not remember any instance where AL displayed "very odd behavior," but noted that AL did seem to "always be fixing his hair." According to this former student AL "kept cleaning supplies in a black bag, and always kept the bag with him." It wasn't clear if the bag contained school or cleaning supplies. Like other former students, this individual did not recall AL ever talking about guns or violence in any way. He did remember hearing that "AL didn't have any friends before the tech club."

The head of security at the high school was the advisor for the Tech Club and apparently asked some older students to "watch out" for AL because he was a little odd and "very shy." The advisor wanted the other students to help AL socialize more. Former students did not remember AL being bullied or teased, but at least one individual stated that he "wouldn't be surprised if [AL] was bullied or teased at high school."

Additionally, at least one student stated that the Tech Club "really did try to befriend [AL]." Tech Club had "lots of odd members, but AL wasn't that extraordinarily different at that time. He would laugh at the stuff we did or said, would occasionally make jokes with us in Tech Club . . . [AL] seemed to enjoy being with us." AL was observed to attend some of the Tech Club parties and was described by another youth as having a good time.

The Technology Club would broadcast games live on a local channel that the kids called "NTV." AL would sign up to tape games and be the cameraman or help out in other ways. AL would "hang out" in the Tech room at school during his free period, lunch time, and even after school. At least one youth said that AL would sometimes "offer up bits of information . . . or chat about what other youth were talking about." AL was described by some youth as initially shy but later "opening up" to some members of the club. One former student said that he thought of AL as "normal," and that others thought "no different of him than other" kids, even despite knowing that AL had some preoccupations such as not wanting to be touched and sanitizing his hands if you accidentally shook them.

One individual remembered the day that AL told a joke in front of other kids, and everyone "paused and then started laughing because it was a funny joke. We gave him a group hug and he seemed to let us do it without a problem." AL was described as enjoying video games, such as Fantasy Start, an online game, and Pokemon 6. He enjoyed watching animated TV, Japanese films—with or without subtitles—some of which he watched with groups of students in the Tech Room at school.

A few former students noted that the Tech Club advisor had taken him under his wing and asked others to be kind and include him. The advisor was terminated from employment in 2008 and at least one former student speculated that this was the reason AL dropped out of school.

AL and Community College

As stated above, he registered for and took several courses at Norwalk Community College and Western Connecticut State University in 2008 and 2009, many for high school graduation credits.. These classes included "website production" and "Visual Basic" (earning an A- and A, respectively.) In the fall of 2008, AL took Data Modeling and DB Design, withdrawing during the semester, and Introduction to Ethical Theory, for which he earned a C. In the Spring of 2009, he took Introductory German and American History Since 1877, as well as Principles of Macroeconomics.

Email correspondence indicates that AL may have struggled attending community college, unable to concentrate and organize himself, and distraught when he could not maintain himself or hand in work. He was unwilling to follow through and work with a tutor, and according to his mother would sometimes cry and say he couldn't go.

In 2009, AL sought to increase his college class load. His father wrote to him of his concerns:

> As we discussed, we will be working on your study skills in order to better prepare you for your upcoming increased college class load. Teaching post-graduate classes for the last 15 years makes me qualified to coach you.
> I have cc'd your mother on this email and asked that she print it out and place it on the counter. I will continue to include your mother on these emails until such time that you regularly check for, and respond to, emails from me.
> We will review your Math homework this weekend when I am in Newtown. Please complete your Math homework by Friday night at midnight. This deadline is not arbitrary. Learning to set and meet deadlines is a critical factor in time management. Time management in turn, is a key study skill. Over the years I had had a number of students that have encountered problems because they have under estimated the amount of time required to complete their assignments. I find that students who are good at time management always do better than their less disciplined peers. Let me know if you have any questions.
>
> Dad.

AL and His Family

AL's mental condition appeared to deteriorate in later adolescence. He became increasingly constrained by obsessive, compulsive behavior. He was hypersensitive to tactile sensations, and very vulnerable to feeling ill at ease, threatened, and suspicious.

Mrs. Lanza appears to have navigated his disabilities entirely through hypervigilance and management of his symptoms. She wrote to a school staff in 2007 that AL had a bad day and therefore his homework was not complete. She explained that she had "interrupted him" by cooking her dinner the night before, even though she knew the smell of food upset him. She added that a repair man had to come to the house in the morning and that as a result AL was "highly agitated." She said that the staff member should make the day "as smooth as possible," and that she would sit in the car and come if he couldn't tolerate class. On the other hand, she also wrote how important is was for him not to feel that "he is running the show." She seemed to want to set up each day for him as he could handle it, but to ensure that he would not know of any special treatment or accommodation.

To balance the observation that Mrs. Lanza was "placating" AL, it is important to note that she was also struggling to figure out what the best course of support and treatment was for her son, with his strong proscriptions for her behavior and his aversion to therapy and medication. While Mrs. Lanza may have rejected or ultimately dismissed some of the recommendations and opportunities offered by the Yale evaluation, she also grappled with her own emotions regarding the complexities of raising a child with significant needs.

Based on her extensive involvement in his curricular and daily activities Mrs. Lanza was attempting to eliminate as many distractions and disruptions to his routine as possible. Also, it is clear throughout that Mrs. Lanza was often at a loss regarding how to get AL to attend school or go to tutoring. In some of her e-mails she paints a picture of desperation and indicates that she does not know what to do - perhaps leading her to placate and appease AL.

The following email exchange is an important reflection of the status of AL's relationship with his mother in his teenage years and their dynamic of mutual dependency.

August 2008 (AL is 16 years old, 11th grade): Email from AL to His mother, 11:25 p.m.

> You do not seem to understand that I was attempting to comfort you with what I consider to be a maxim with which to live. You unfortunately probably still do not understand what I mean. As a disclaimer: I type nothing in this that is in a tone that is condescending, vindictive, malicious, snide, malignant, or any synonym that you can think of. I mean well.
>
> If you believe that you wasted your life, as you seem to have insinuated, you will gain nothing from regretting it and will only depress yourself; you cannot change anything from the past. There is something that I can assure you of that will always be true: it does not matter if you live for the next one year, five years, ten years, fifteen years, twenty years, thirty years, fifty years or even 100 years; the day before you die you will regret ever worrying about your life instead of thinking of what you want to do.
>
> Every new year that you do live, you will regret not having started anything that you wanted to do the year prior, only regretting the past more.
>
> What I mean is that you should think of what you want to do today; not starting next year or next month, but today. Thinking that you are not going to be able to do anything in the future will only ensure that fate. Also thinking that you are too "old" is going to ensure the same fate.
>
> It is not as though I do not mean that you are homeless and begging; I would spend my life savings to prevent that out of obligation for what you have done for me. My personality is merely inherently unmoving; I will not be upset over

something that you cannot change. And you should not be upset either. What you should do is think about what you want to do.

I also want to mention that I purchased something two weeks ago on Newegg to double your computer's memory without even saying anything until now. I do not try to avoid doing anything for you as you seem to think. I am glad that I was born, and I appreciate your having taken care of me. (It is not my fault if you have not detected as much of an increase in speed as I would have liked, however; I blame its outdated processor. I would change that if I could, but it's not possible to do so for your model.) Please read the first paragraph again.

Email Response from Mrs. Lanza, 1:05 a.m.

I appreciate your effort to be a comfort to me. I apologize if I seemed angry or antagonistic. I was simply over emotional and as it is often the case worrying about the future. I admit that I have been feeling a bit overwhelmed by my circumstances lately, but in no way do I regret having raised two wonderful children. I have high hopes for you both and will consider my life a success if you and Ryan live happy and productive lives.

There are a few things that I do regret . . . one of the biggest is that I dropped out of college, believing it to be more important to help your father get through college. Financially, it was impossible for us to afford a college education for both of us, and it seemed more important that he receive a diploma. In some ways I regret leaving the workforce as it has severely limited my prospects for the future, but again, it was a decision that I made to take more responsibility for the house and the children, and to allow your father to concentrate on his career. I do feel that I was able to be a better mother and have been able to put great effort into raising you and your brother, so that regret is mitigated in that respect. On the occasion that Ryan or you show some appreciation for my efforts, I feel completely justified in that choice and dually rewarded.

I know that it is harder for you to show appreciation, and that it does not come as a natural response. I really do not want you to feel obligated in that way. I do not expect any help, financial or otherwise, from you or your brother, and would not accept it if it were offered. I am certain that I will not be homeless or begging on a street corner, as your father is obligated by law and morality to see that my 30 years of service and sacrifice are compensated for. He has assured me that I will live a comfortable life and that my health expenses are covered. He is an honorable man. I am grateful that I was married to someone who honors his responsibilities. He has also taking [sic] responsibility to provide a college education for both you and your brother, so that neither of you will have to struggle and sacrifice as we did.

If you choose to, you will emerge from college with a master's degree of your choice, debt free, to pursue any career in life that you wish. When I think of what I would like to do for the future, I think I would like to get my college degree first. I just thought of that tonight, as a direct result of my conversation with you. I think it would be possible as I dropped out only a year shy of my degree, and it seems as I might be spending quite a bit of time on campus waiting for you to take classes, so why not take advantage of that?! I suppose I could take classes at the same time you are taking classes.

I agree with you when you say that I should try to think positively of the future and what I want to do today. There is nothing that I can do about my diagnosis, and I do try to be as healthy as I can, despite the prognosis. I am sure that you noticed that I exercise regularly and do my best to stay in good shape. It's not like I have the attitude that since I will be crippled anyway I may as well give up and get fat and sedentary now. I am working hard to stay as healthy as I can, for as long as I can.

At some point, I might like to start a business. I sometimes toy with the idea of an internet business like my friend, [L], owns. (Did I punctuate that last sentence correctly?) Her website is [xxx]. You should have a look at it sometime and let me know what you think of it.

Anyway, I would like you to know that no matter what, I am very proud of the person you are. I have no preconceived notion of how you should react or respond. I know that you tend to be more reserved and less emotional and I do not perceive that as condescending malignant, or callous. You are pragmatic and stoical. These are fine attributes. I am glad to know that you are glad to be born and appreciate being taken care of. I love you very much and am more than happy to take care of you in any way I can. I suppose I have felt that you didn't even notice how hard I try to make things as tolerable as possible for you and that has made me feel sad in a way. I am much happier now, knowing that you do not despise me for bringing you into this world. Above all, I want you to be happy, no matter what you choose to do.

You may not think I notice, but my computer is working faster and I have been able to download bank statements faster and search the websites quicker. I was able to get baseball scores for all the games in a split second, and watch a video clip that a friend sent without any freezing. I didn't know that you had worked on it, so I thank you for your efforts. You should let me know when you do thoughtful things so that you can get credit! As an aside, I am having a problem that has been ongoing for months. The cursor abruptly moves to a different place in text now and again when I am in the middle of typing a sentence. It is very strange and annoying. Maybe you can have a look at it sometime? Thank you for taking the time to send me this e-mail. I now understand your motive and meaning, and I truly appreciate it!

Mr. Lanza appeared to defer most parental decision-making and responsibility regarding educational, medical, and mental health issues to Mrs. Lanza. His statement to police that Mrs. Lanza thought "homeschooling" AL would be best is indicative of the deference Mr. Lanza exhibited for Mrs.

Lanza's decisions. Mr. Lanza is not mentioned or identified in any of the medical records, and is only noted to be present for educational IEP meetings in 2007.

In an interview with journalist Andrew Solomon for the New Yorker Magazine, Mr. Lanza described the routines and complexities of his life with AL[85]. For years, even after the parents' separation, Mr. Lanza saw AL regularly, taking him and his brother for weekend hikes and other activities. The two talked about politics, history, and other significant themes. Mr. Lanza described AL as talkative and having a "sharp sense of humor."[86]

From 2009 to 2010, tensions seemed to escalate for AL and the family. By 2009, AL's parents had divorced. According to Mrs. Lanza, AL said that he did not want to see his father anymore. It is not clear whether he really said that or if that was his mother's interpretation of his wishes. Over the next few years, continuing until the weeks before December 14, 2012, Mr. Lanza would email invitations to AL, trying to entice him to go hiking or do other activities together. AL never responded. Mr. Lanza did not understand what was impeding AL's response, or what, if anything, he could do to engage his increasingly impossible-to reach son. He thought about showing up at the house, but felt that given Mrs. Lanza's concern about maintaining order and predictability for AL, that neither she nor his son would welcome this approach. He also thought about hiring a private investigator so that he could run in to AL in the community, but this plan didn't seem to make much sense either. He thought perhaps he could wait it out, that time would heal the relationship, or that eventually he could entice AL into seeing him.

Firearms and Mental Illness

AL grew up in a home where it was common place to use guns for recreational activity. It cannot be overlooked that as his mental health deteriorated and his isolation from the world increased dramatically, his access to guns did not diminish. His parents, and certainly his mother, seemed unaware of any potential detrimental impact of providing unfettered access to firearms to their son. Particularly in the waning months of AL's life, when his mother noted that he would not leave the house and seemed despondent, it is not clear that she took measures to curtail his access to guns or whether she considered his potential for suicide or other acts of violence. Additionally, there is no mention of access to or use of firearms in any other available educational, medical, or mental health records.

In later interviews with state police, Mr. Lanza indicated that he had never given or purchased a firearm for AL but that he assumed Mrs. Lanza had. Mr. Lanza indicated that he was unaware that Mrs. Lanza was buying AL his own guns, as opposed to simply doing shooting activities together. Mr. Lanza indicated he knew AL had access to guns when he took him to a shooting range and AL had two long guns that Mr. Lanza believed were purchased by Mrs. Lanza.

---

[85] Solomon, *supra* note 34, at 6.
[86] *Id.occ*

Records and interviews indicate that the Lanza family owned firearms over the years and regularly participated in activities at local shooting ranges. The family engaged in shooting activities with the children from a young age. AL and his mother took the basic NRA rifle safety course. AL, per police interviews, first engaged in recreational shooting activities at age 5 with his family.

Mr. Lanza indicated that on several occasions prior to 2010 he took AL to a local shooting range. They would rent a single gun to shoot at targets, and Mr. Lanza would purchase ammunition at the shooting range for the two of them to use. Mr. Lanza said that on every occasion, he always kept the unused ammunition and he never let AL keep ammunition for himself.

As stated earlier in this report, the focus of this review is not primarily on the role of guns and their relationship to violence or mass murder. However, given the questions that have been asked in the wake of this tragedy and the issues raised regarding access to guns for the mentally ill, authors offer a few observations regarding the relationship between guns, mental illness, and violent acts.

While the prevalence of severe mental illness is roughly stable around the world, for instance the prevalence of schizophrenia is approximately 1% in all developed countries,[87] the rates of gun violence vary widely and are generally in keeping with the prevalence of guns in various societies. In other words, while millions of people in the developed world may have schizophrenia, only an infinitesimal number of those individuals will engage in acts of violence. But rates of gun violence around the world do vary widely based on access to guns.

"A widely cited 2010 study in the American Journal of Law & Economics showed that gun-related homicides in Australia dropped 59% between 1995 and 2006. The firearm-suicide rate dropped 65%."[88] This was after meaningful gun control regulations which outlawed possession of assault weapons were passed following a mass shooting. Great Britain has also shown a marked reduction in gun crimes since instituting a hand gun ban following a mass school shooting which occurred in 1996.[89]

The conclusion that access to guns drives shooting episodes far more than the presence of mental illness is inescapable. Those countries that have tight gun controls in general experience less overall gun violence and have fewer episodes per capita of mass shootings.

Further, there is good reason to believe that the nearly ubiquitous presence of assault weapons and high capacity bullet clips enhances the number of individuals likely to be shot in shooting incidents. We also know that the period during which a shooter must reload provides an opportunity for others

---

[87] *Burden of Mental Illness*, CENTER FOR DISEASE CONTROL AND PREVENTION, http://www.cdc.gov/mentalhealth/basics/burden.htm (last visited Nov. 3, 2014).
[88] *Gun Violence Panel, Before the Senate Judiciary Comm.*, 113th Cong. 1 (2013) (testimony of Dr. William Begg, Director, Emergency Medical Services, Danbury Hospital, Danbury Connecticut), *available at* http://www.judiciary.senate.gov/download/testimony-of-begg-pdf. (*citing* Leigh, A., Neill, C., *Do Gun Buybacks Save Lives? Evidence from Panel Data*, 12 AM. L. AND ECON. REV. 509, 518 (2010)).
[89] M.J. North, *Gun Control in Great Britain after the Dunblane Shootings, in* REDUCING GUN VIOLENCE IN AMERICA: INFORMING POLICY WITH EVIDENCE AND ANALYSIS 185, 189–92 (D.W. & J.S. Vernick eds., 2013).

to stop the shooter or to escape. Jared Loughner's massacre in Tuscon, Arizona ended only when, after emptying a 33 round magazine, killing and wounding another, he was subdued by bystanders while attempting to exchange magazines. In Sandy Hook Elementary School, eleven children escaped from their classroom while AL was exchanging the clip in his automatic weapon. The smaller the capacity of the clip, the more reloading episodes there will be, and the greater the opportunity for escape or rescue by law enforcement.

It is reasonable to wonder what actions AL would have taken and whether the Sandy Hook tragedy could have occurred at all if he had not had unfettered access to significant weaponry and ammunition.

SUMMARY AND RECOMMENDATIONS: AGES 14 THROUGH 18

If there is a single document that is most prescient regarding AL's deterioration, it is the October 2006 report from the Yale Child Study Center—an evaluation that so dramatically states the high stakes presented by AL's disabilities and the need for meaningful and immediate intervention.

Appropriate, multidisciplinary and expert treatment, integrated into the family setting, community, and school might have prevented the later deterioration in AL's mental state. The lack of sustained, expert-driven and well-coordinated mental health treatment, and medical and educational planning ultimately enabled his progressive deterioration. Though again, no direct line of causation can be drawn from these failures to his commission of mass murder.

AL's school district did not—or was not able to—meet his needs for individual education planning. The team, including Mrs. Lanza, became focused on curricular issues to the exclusion of AL's developmental and mental health needs. Though one of his school evaluators urgently noted that the curriculum was *not* the problem, the school allowed itself to become very and singularly focused on the academic content of AL's day. Despite his profound and increasing school-phobia and school refusals, there was no development or mention of a Functional Behavioral Assessment or Behavioral Intervention Plan to address the phobias, aversions and social anxieties that AL presented with[90]. The records reflect a near complete absence of attention to social-emotional learning. The Individual Education Plans simply do not address this profound and central need.

Authors do not conclude that the educational team was indifferent to AL's needs or goals. Rather, the school district and AL's family appeared very invested in AL's success and greatly desired him to graduate high school and attend college. However, they did not pursue the multidisciplinary and expert treatment for AL's severe emotional disturbance that had been recommended by both the Danbury Hospital and Yale psychiatric evaluations in 2005-2006. Additionally, the educational planning demonstrates a lack of knowledge of or adherence to regulatory requirements and best practices.

---

[90]Special Education Law requires the development of a Functional Behavioral Assessment and Functional Behavioral Intervention Plan when a child's behavior impedes his or her learning.

Both AL's mother and his educational team shared a goal of managing and accommodating, rather than securing treatment for, AL's disabilities, and likely this approach was fueled by a lack of critical information and guidance. This approach may also have been supported by input, at least initially, from the community psychiatrist, though later school records contain no updated mental health information. The father's earlier efforts to ensure care coordination and effective information sharing seemed not to have had lasting effect. The documentary and interview evidence indicates that AL's emotional disturbance and social isolation improved at most a small amount and only transiently, leaving him significantly debilitated as he transitioned out of secondary school.

Schools may often operate without the all of the information from community providers, and may not have multi-disciplinary therapeutic experts on staff. Here there is little documentation of what efforts were made to ensure appropriate expertise and care coordination was brought to bear on the educational planning process.

Is there a Reluctance to Serve Youths' Social-Emotional Learning Needs in School?

There is great variance in the ability and activity of schools in evaluating, identifying, and addressing the social-emotional and developmental needs of children with disabilities. Social Emotional, developmental, and behavioral health needs are sometimes considered parenthetical to the learning process. It is not uncommon for schools not to have a social worker or other therapeutic support staff in the building. It is also not uncommon for an Individual Education Plan to refer to social-emotional or mental health needs and indicate that those needs are being met in the community by an outpatient provider.

It is imperative to note that federal special education laws *require* districts to identify students with social-emotional and developmental challenges that impede educational progress and that educational plans must include research-based interventions and supports to meet individual students' needs.[91] The law also requires that progress towards identified goals be carefully documented.[92]

But because schools may not be equipped to provide, or even to import, comprehensive behavioral health or developmental supports to children, precious services or expertise are tightly rationed so that districts can serve many children with their allotted resources. It is not uncommon for special education and related services to be downsized as districts face resource-conscious budgets.

AL's condition presented further challenges in this regard as he struggled with both developmental challenges consistent with an Autism Spectrum Disorder and mental health challenges associated with Obsessive Compulsive Disorder, anxiety and a preoccupation with violence. The compounding effect of multiple diagnoses, combined with a preoccupation with violence, would have raised significant complexities for any treatment.[93]

---

[91] 20 U.S.C. § 1411(e)(2)(C) (2013); 34 C.F.R. § 300.34 (2014) (obligations to use scientific and research-based instruction and evaluation strategies); 34 C.F.R § 300.304 (2014) (obligation to evaluate in all areas of disability).
[92] 34 C.F.R. § 300.347(a)(2) (2014).
[93] S. Logan, et al., *Rates and Predictors of Adherence to Psychotropic Medications in Children with Autism Spectrum Disorders*, 44 J. OF AUTISM AND DEVELOPMENTAL DISORDERS 2931–48 (2014).

Multiple Treatment or Service Providers Were Involved with AL and His Family, But There was No Clear Coordination of Care or Transition Planning

Records analysis reveals some of the "right" things happening for AL, at least early on in school and the community. His mother consulted with his pediatrician on various aspects of his well-being. He received some clinical support from a psychiatrist, and he had an active and engaged Individual Education Planning team in his local school district. AL was seen for evaluation and treatment recommendations at the Yale Child Study Center, and Mr. and Mrs. Lanza made efforts to try and incorporate feedback from multiple providers into the educational planning process. However, these systems: school, pediatrics, and out-patient mental health, were not able to effectively or clearly communicate with each other. *The records from the Yale Child Study Center and the community psychiatrist are notably not present in AL's school record, and the educational recommendations from Yale are not referenced in or imbedded into AL's IEP.* Partly as a result of this dearth of integrated information and expertise, when efforts to "mainstream" AL failed, the team (including AL's parents) reverted back to creating the "prosthetic" environment that the Child Study Center cautioned against.

The dynamics presented here are not unique to this educational team, these parents, or this school district, but rather reflect with systemic concerns over siloed systems of education, physical health, and mental health care for children. When adults sit at the treatment planning or educational planning table to discuss how best to serve a child and his family, the question must always be asked: do we have the right people here and what more do we need to know in order to make a decision that is truly in the best interests of the child? Therapeutic and other related services must be readily available in schools and communities and the expertise easily shared amongst providers.

Notably, present-day interviews with some school personnel provided their perspective that in making so many individualized accommodations for AL, they in fact adequately responded to his social-emotional needs, helping him learn in the only way he could given his significant anxiety and emotional problems. These individuals opined that there is only so much a school can do, and they do what they can to focus on education in the context of a child's mental health problems. The problem for AL, according to some personnel, was that after he graduated and had to do without his IEP team, there was nothing in the community for him to receive, and that the true systemic problem is the lack of appropriate supports for young adults with mental health problems.

These observations reflect common perspective and practice in schools and are certainly correct regarding the dearth of appropriate services for young adults with mental health and developmental disorders. However, this perspective also underestimates school districts' obligations and ability to offer comprehensive, multidisciplinary supports via school resources and coordination with community services, including state agencies that serve disabled adolescents and young adults. The law and best practice standards provide that such coordination and support must continue until a youth's 21st birthday if so needed. The fact that AL was unable to function post-graduation is, in part, a reflection of the lack of community services for young adults, but is also due to the lack of sustained and effective transition planning and the IEP team's agreement to graduate AL early.

AL's Family Relationships and Psychological State in Adolescence

Over the years, AL's parents had difficulty engaging AL with sustained or appropriate mental health and developmental support services. Mrs. Lanza struggled with her intuitive urge to protect AL from any discomfort and his growing need for evaluation and intervention. Her choices over the years highlight how a parent's desire to see her child in a positive light and protect him from distress can inadvertently lead to assumptions and decisions that are not in the child's best interests.

Though Mrs. Lanza brought AL to Danbury Hospital in 2005 during an apparent mental health crisis, she did not allow him to be fully evaluated or treated, later recounting that she felt making him stay in the hospital was "abuse." But this protective instinct resulted in her refusing the very help he needed to address his severe distress. Mrs. Lanza's primary interest at the time was in continuing to manage AL's fear. She was not looking for treatment options from emergency department staff. She wanted to get him home and keep him home.

Of the couple of providers that saw AL, only one—the Yale Child Study Center— seemed to appreciate the gravity of AL's presentation, his need for extensive mental health and special education supports, and the critical need for medication to ease his obsessive-compulsive symptoms. It was Mr. Lanza that seemed the most willing to push AL to take the medication and align himself with the provider's recommendations. Almost immediately after medication was prescribed and taken, Mrs. Lanza contacted the provider to state that AL would no longer take it. Although the main side effect complained of by the family was not attributable to the prescribed medication, and although the provider took pains to explain the potential benefit of the medication, the decision was made to discontinue it.

> In the course of AL's entire life, minimal mental health evaluation and treatment (in relation to his apparent need) was ever obtained.

Ultimately, Mrs. Lanza determined that it was not productive for AL to continue with the Yale Child Study Center—preferring to keep AL with the community psychiatrist whose therapeutic contribution remains unknown. What can be gleaned from authors' review is that the community psychiatrist seemed more aligned with Mrs. Lanza's desire to accommodate AL's disabilities and predilections, and was less likely to challenge AL and push him out of his comfort zone. Mrs. Lanza admitted that she instinctively prioritized AL's comfort, maybe to the detriment of other needs.

Some of the failure to engage AL with effective treatment was likely due to his reluctance or refusal to engage with these providers. According to records, AL disagreed with his Asperger's diagnosis and did not see the benefit of individual therapy. By a certain age, it may have been difficult to compel AL to physically leave the house, get in a car, and be transported somewhere he did not want to go. According to Mrs. Lanza he "loathed" the clinician at Yale and did not see the benefit of going. It may have seemed better to assuage him and hope progress could be made elsewhere. Notably, authors review of payment records to the community psychiatrist suggest that AL's contact with this provider ended even as his mental health issues seemed to worsen from 2008 onward.

The records present a theme of attempting to shield and protect AL from stress yet simultaneously making decisions for him which reduced his ability to benefit from contacts with peers and the outside world. Mrs. Lanza's middle-of-the-night email to AL in 2008 speaks to the great lengths she went to set things up for him in a way that would cause him the least stress, an effort she hoped he

83

had or would appreciate. It also shows how freely she shared her own anxieties and resentments with AL, as if he were an adult who could be a close confidante, and his response suggests that this may have been well beyond his relatively immature emotional capacities.

Mrs. Lanza appeared to be a major factor, likely unwitting, in increasing AL's isolation from the world. She padded his world and shielded him, even from landscapers that visited the home. She described "peeking in [AL's] room," and hoping that he would not find out about it. Mr. Lanza did not appreciate how detrimental this dynamic was or know how to alter it. He ultimately deferred to Mrs. Lanza's judgment regarding management of AL's educational plan and mental health treatment.

Efforts made by Mrs. Lanza not to infringe on AL's sensibilities had some impact. But the effort to create an artificial bubble added to his isolation, which only grew deeper after high school. Despite some gains for AL in high school and his social affiliation with the Technology Club, his parents permitted him to withdraw from the high school environment again. Later, Mrs. Lanza affirmatively told Mr. Lanza that AL would not visit with him and she effectively discouraged Mr. Lanza from coming to engage him.

While most families of children with autism or mental health disorders collaborate with school and treatment teams, it is not uncommon to find ambivalence around accepting help. In many cases, the child can communicate and presents without grossly atypical behavior and so the parents struggle to accept and embrace a diagnosis like autism. In some families, other life issues or parental mental health issues take precedence and impede follow-through with educational and clinical recommendations. In the most difficult cases, the parents who are conflicted over having the child grow up and become independent or who enjoy attention from providers and teachers, can consciously and unconsciously sabotage efforts that would facilitate development.[94] However, school districts need to acknowledge that relying solely on parent reports to inform educational plans can have long lasting detrimental effects on a child's education. More work needs to be done to allow various providers in a child's life to communicate and collaborate.

As AL appeared to become progressively more isolated from peers and adults (other than relatively superficial relationships, e.g., attending community college classes and completing classwork for instructors), his family relationships seemed to be either similarly detached (i.e., making no response to his father's occasional invitations and no evidence of contact with his brother) or a mix of emotional detachment and instances of distant and confused, but apparently sincere attempts to communicate emotional caring (with his mother, as exemplified by the pair of lengthy e-mails between them in 2008).

Mr. Lanza recounts how he was told late in AL's adolescence that AL did not want to visit with him anymore—a sentiment conveyed second hand through AL's mother. The distance and alleged refusal went on for two years, according to Mr. Lanza. Mr. Lanza indicated that he did not know how to

---

[94] Harris, S.L. and Powers, M.D. (1984) Behavior therapists look at the impact of an autistic child on the family system. In E. Schopler and G Mesibov (Eds.) The effects of autism on the family. New York: Plenum; Powers, M.D. and Thorwath, C.A. (1988) Treating the family system. In M.D. Powers (Ed.) Expanding systems of service delivery for persons with developmental disabilities. Baltimore: Paul H. Brookes.

bridge the distance, though he tried many strategies including offering to buy AL a computer, presenting favored outings and other incentives, and even demanding to set an expectation that AL would see him. Ultimately, Mr. Lanza decided he could not simply show up at the house uninvited. Mrs. Lanza often indicated that she would try to convince AL to see his father but that he would steadfastly refuse.

The emails between AL and his mother in late 2008 suggest that he was genuinely attempting to express caring and sympathy for his mother, both through his words (to which she responds with appreciation in her e-mail back to him) and actions in the best way that he can think of, by helping to make her computer more efficient. AL and Mrs. Lanza's email exchanges show his limitations and eventual deterioration in social-emotional functioning.

The email exchanges show a dynamic of mutual dependency and a somewhat parentified role for AL. The use of emails to communicate shows his preference for maintaining some distance from Mrs. Lanza (as he eventually seems to do with most of his contacts with other people). Mrs. Lanza spoke to AL about her concern about becoming destitute, physically incapacitated or otherwise seriously afflicted, her sacrifice and struggle for AL, her unfulfilled aspirations for herself, and very significantly, showing her love for him by trying to make life "tolerable for him." Mrs. Lanza's efforts to make life "tolerable" for AL often involved, in the Yale Child Study Center psychiatrist's prescient words, "adapting the world to AL, rather than helping him to adapt to the world." Despite AL's continued and escalating struggles later in high school and after graduation, there is no indication of any other attempt by either parent to resume or identify treatment services.

Was Deference to the Family's Decision-Making Appropriate?

A review of AL's history raises questions regarding whether any providers, particularly the educational system and pediatrics, viewing a youth with profound developmental and mental health challenges, who was at times borderline or actually anorexic, and who was often unavailable for school or treatment, considered that AL's parents needed assistance or otherwise lacked capacity to ensure that his specialized needs were met.

In Connecticut, all of the providers who worked with AL were mandated reporters of suspected child abuse *or* neglect. A mandatory reporter must report any child who he or she "reasonably suspects" may be a victim of abuse or neglect.[95] In Connecticut, a child may be deemed neglected if he or she "is being denied proper care and attention, physically, educationally, emotionally or morally."[96]

Making a referral regarding suspected abuse or neglect to a child welfare agency can be a daunting proposition. Additionally, the ability of a child welfare agency, possibly mistrusted by a parent, caregiver, or even provider, to ably engage a reluctant parent or child into mental health services may be very limited.

Crafting a state agency response to a caregiver who seems unable to ensure the specialized needs of a child are met—*even for understandable or protective reasons*-- necessitates an institutional capacity to assess

---

[95] Conn. Gen. Stat. § 17a-101.
[96] Conn. Gen. Stat. §46b-120.

why the caregiver or family system is struggling and how the family will best be engaged and stay engaged. The role of a child welfare system may inevitably be to compel a family into support services, a role that may, admittedly bring with it suspicion or fear on the part of the child or family.

However, it is fair to query here whether the Lanzas, after all engagement with community mental health services ended, needed to be compelled into services and whether this type of action may have arrested AL's deterioration and isolation from the community. Or whether, at a minimum, Mr. Lanza—who did not have the same access or direct knowledge of AL's presentation as Mrs. Lanza--needed to be drawn further into the educational and mental health planning with providers at that time.

Should a formal red flag have gone up regarding the family's ability to meet AL's specialized needs, particularly after 10th grade when AL remained unable to attend school, markedly underweight and unwilling to attend or otherwise unengage with treatment?

Surely the providers encountering this family could understand the parents' concerns, confusion, and lack of understanding of the scope or magnitude of their child's problems. Providers may have also understood and had compassion for the parents' reluctance to pursue certain types of treatment strategies for their child, who himself appeared anxious and resistant to medication and therapy, despite how helpful or necessary it might have been.

Looking at the pediatric record, the pediatrician knew that AL had significant diagnoses, was losing weight (at times), anxious, obsessive compulsive, had repetitive hand washing that led to excoriation, experienced numerous somatic and probably psychosomatic complaints, and was not attending school with his peers. The pediatrician knew that AL was, for a time at least, seeing a psychiatrist in the community, though there is no indication that the doctor had information from this mental health provider or knew what the frequency and duration of this service was.

The doctor also seemed to know that despite his recommendation for a neurological consultation, none appeared to take place, as the doctor received no updates or reports from a specialist. Certainly, as stated earlier, this information was enough to warrant careful follow-up and care coordination from the pediatrician. There is no documentation of efforts by the pediatrician to engage this family with appropriate and *sustained* mental health care. There is also no indication in the record of the pediatrician's recognition of the significance of AL's presentation. Indeed, if the significance of AL's condition went unrecognized, it is likely that the doctor would not have had concerns about the capacity of the parent to meet his needs. It is not uncommon to have relatively little communication between a primary care provider and a mental health specialist unless the primary care provider has recognized that she has a problem before her for which she feels the need for expert assistance.

Similar issues are raised in the context of AL's schooling from 2008 onward. While there was initial extensive parental involvement, particularly by Mr. Lanza in 2007, to ensure information-sharing and care coordination between the school and community mental health providers, by the end of 10th grade, AL was again unable to attend high school classes and was no longer engaged in mental health treatment. While AL enrolled in college classes for high school credit, this was purportedly because his anxiety prevented him from attending high school.

It is not clear what steps the school district took, beyond correspondence in the spring of 2006 (AL's 8th grade), to confirm or determine what treatment was in fact being provided to AL or his family. However, it is also possible that school personnel may have asked for and received verbal updates from Mrs. Lanza that *do not appear in the school* record, and the answers the school received were satisfactory.

It appeared that AL's functioning and mental status continued to deteriorate, leaving him less and less able to participate in a "free and appropriate public education." Concurrently, the school should have noted or asked questions about how AL's need for an appropriate education could possibly be met by at times his prolonged "independent study" status, particularly given the district's legal obligation to craft and offer an educational plan that addressed all aspects of AL's disabilities.

The reluctance to take an adversarial posture with a family that is invested and concerned with their child's welfare can certainly be understood. But educational providers are also mandatory reporters of suspected neglect and if a district has information that the needs of a child are not or cannot be met by his caregiver, these reporters are obligated to bring this to the attention of the child welfare system. In this case, authors cannot know the degree to which Mrs. Lanza may have heightened or mollified the school's concerns about AL, and she certainly presented as invested and concerned for his welfare. The overall impression school professionals had was of a concerned and engaged parent who knew how to manage her son's unique needs.

Individuals can, of course, disagree as to whether AL's parents' decision to permit him to stay home or attend tutoring rather than attend school and the decision to stop pursuing mental health treatment after 10th grade falls under the category of decisions that parents are free to make regardless of outside disagreement. But individuals may also conclude here that to be presented with a youth with profound and chronic disabilities who was removed systematically *(or permitted to remove himself)* from opportunities for treatment and education, raised a reasonable basis for concern regarding the capacity of his caregivers to meet his needs, and that additional steps should have been taken.

School teams and clinical providers face a dilemma when considering a referral to a child welfare agency related to a failure to follow through with needed treatment. Upon making the referral, the family may cut off contact and so the provider loses the opportunity to continue efforts to deliver needed treatment. Additionally, with the importance of confidentiality, it may be hard to ascertain if the family is working with other providers. Even with the case of AL, it would have been difficult to predict the risk of violence and the tragic outcome, and the family could possibly have made a credible case that they believed that they were meeting his needs.

Mrs. Lanza, and early on in high school Mr. Lanza as well, presented as invested and caring about AL's educational experience, thus increasing the likelihood that school professionals may have wanted to partner with her and that they would have deferred to her judgment about what was best for him. Additionally, Mrs. Lanza consistently indicated to school personnel that AL wanted to be treated as a "regular student."

Would a similar family from a different race or lower socio-economic status in the community have been given the same benefit of the doubt that AL's family was given? Is the community more reluctant to intervene and more likely to provide deference to the parental judgment and decision-making of white, affluent parents than those caregivers who are poor or minority?[97] Would AL's caregivers' reluctance to maintain him in school or a treatment program have gone under the radar if he were a child of color?

These questions are meant for reflection, rather than blame, as we must grapple with the issues of how our systems assess families' needs, alternately red flagging, or supporting families and children from different races and backgrounds. These issues also point to the need for further development of models to use in the child protection system so that families may be better engaged with effective treatment.

Did Helping Systems Offer the Right Help?

To balance the observations regarding Mrs. Lanza's rejection of certain treatment or educational options, it is useful to consider what types of supports were offered to the family over time. Whether AL received the right help is critical to understanding whether the trajectory of his mental health deterioration and eventual complete isolation could have been altered. This is not the same as concluding that but for a particular action on behalf of an individual or provider, the shootings would not have happened.

Through hindsight, authors can see that AL and his family did not get all of the right help early on, long before Mrs. Lanza began *rejecting or failing to seek out certain types of help*. Again, we note that it is not uncommon for parents to vacillate between acknowledging and denying their child's need for services. All children are a little different from each other, and gauging whether a child's differences are in need of outside intervention or special attention at any given stage of development can be daunting to determine.

Here, it is not clear whether the school system or AL's pediatrician, while perhaps noting that AL struggled with anxiety, social phobias, fitting in, and eventually powerful fears about being in school, offered AL or his parents a vision of how various resources could help them. When AL seemed unable to return to school from his homebound status, it was ultimately Mr. Lanza that pursued a referral and recommendations from the Yale Child Study Center, a support group in the community,

---

[97] Research tells us that issues of race and class may affect virtually every aspect of how the state or local actors respond to questions regarding an adult guardian's ability to care for and meet the needs of a child. *See, e.g.,* J Ryan, et al., *Is There a Link Between Child Welfare and Disproportionate Minority Contact in Juvenile Justice, A Knowledge Brief: MacArthur Foundation's Models for Change Research Initiative* (2011); S. Chibnall, et al., *Children of Color in the Child Welfare System: Perspectives from the Child Welfare Community*, CHILDREN'S BUREAU, CHILD INFORMATION GATEWAY (2003).

88

and a private therapeutic program and the development of a well-coordinated Individualized Education Plan.

There is no indication that the school system or the pediatrician effectively coordinated with available service providers or pressed any of the issues regarding AL's mental health and therapeutic needs, nor is there clear indication that school professionals knew what to do about these needs on their own.

Separately, the local hospital emergency department and the Yale Child Study Center were in a better position to offer a plan of action for the family. Here, it appears that a plan of medication management and therapy was offered to AL, and an attempt was made to educate both he and his parents regarding the profound nature of his disability and prognosis and the ways that therapy and medication could help him. The Lanzas' rejection of this plan in favor of working with the community psychiatrist and permitting AL to pursue a high school education largely consisting of tutoring and independent study may look like "non-compliance" to some observers, but may also be the product of genuine confusion regarding his needs and how best to meet them.

Moreover, given AL's apparent intense fears regarding lack of structure or even leaving the house, it is fair to ask what services might have been available to him in the home or in places in the community that he felt comfortable. Given the difficulties of forcing an adolescent to get in a car and travel to a destination that he doesn't want to go, even a therapeutic one, the benefits of home or natural-setting based services seem important to consider. It was the Yale Child Study Center psychiatrist that wrote a cautionary email emphasizing that clinic-based support, without intensive family work and provision of services in the course of AL's daily routine, was unlikely to be successful. While that assessment was apt it cannot be overstated that there remains an extremely limited availability of home and community-based services, particularly for individuals with Autism Spectrum Disorders and co-morbid mental illness *and their families.*

Finally, though special education services are highly focused on the individual child, parents often require additional services in the forms of psycho-education, training and peer-to-peer supports to help them cope and respond to the stressful situations that are coupled with raising a child with special needs. It is unclear if the Lanzas were ever offered this type of support.

The Necessity of Effective Family Engagement Strategies

It is imperative to consider that *many families* struggle to understand their child's mental illness and effectively identify and engage with mental health treatment. Here, AL exhibited reluctance to accept treatment; his mother, and perhaps his father as well, were both interested in and, at times, ambivalent about available treatment options, and eventually these values and concerns may have contributed to AL's ultimate disengagement from support.

Studies show that this is a common problem, and that sometimes those individuals with the most significant conditions may even be more likely to "drop out" of treatment.[98] A family's failure to follow through with support services is also not uncommon even in the wake of the family *initiating* a request for help, which is often the case in AL's story. [99]

Successful, *ongoing* family engagement strategies are critical to effective delivery of services for children. Obstacles to treatment may include everything from the practical—namely, transportation, timing of appointments, and cost—to fundamental differences with family values or a concern regarding the perceived benefit of the treatment offered and the perception of stigma which surrounds mental health treatment.

Studies suggest addressing family engagement as a matter of course may set the foundation of a successful treatment strategy and will be most effective in increasing the family's likelihood to participate in and follow treatment recommendations.[100]

> At different stages of treatment, when new themes emerge or different interaction patterns are targeted for change, new barriers to retention can emerge in different family members. Keeping the family members engaged at these points in the therapy process requires the same thought and skill required early in treatment.[101]

It is also useful to consider what it means for a family to be "engaged" in services. As one researcher writes:

> Engagement is often synonymous with involvement. Involvement of families in child welfare services is important, but real engagement goes beyond that. Families can be involved and compliant without being engaged. Engagement is about motivating and empowering families to recognize their own needs, strengths, and resources, and to take an active role in changing things for the better. Engagement is what keeps families working in the long and sometimes slow process of positive change.[102]

---

[98] E. Ingoldsby, *Review of Interventions to Improve Family Engagement and Retention in Parent and Child Mental Health Programs*, 19 J. CHILD FAM. STUD. 629, 629–45 (2010) (*citing* G.E. Miller GE & R.J. Prinz, *Enhancement of Social Learning Family Interventions for Child Conduct Disorder*, 108 PSYCHOLOGICAL BULLETIN, 291, 291–307 (1990)); J. Snell-Johns, et al., *Evidence-based Solutions for Overcoming Access Barriers, Decreasing Attrition, and Promoting Chance with Underserved Families*. 18 J. OF FAM. PSYCH. 19, 19–35 (2004).

[99] Erin Ingoldsby, *Review of Interventions to Improve Family Engagement and Retention in Parent and Child Mental Health Programs*, 19 J. CHILD FAM. STUD. 629, 629–45 (2010).

[100] *Id.*

[101] N. Chovil, *Engaging Families in Child & Youth Mental Health: A Review of Best, Emerging and Promising Practices*, FAMILY ENGAGEMENT: REVIEW OF LITERATURE 1, 10 (2009) (quoting J.D. Coatsworth, et al., *Brief Strategic Family Therapy versus Community Control: Engagement, Retention, and an Exploration of the Moderating Role of Adolescent Symptom Severity*, 40 J. OF FAM. PROCESS 313–32 (2001)).

[102] *Id.* at 6 (*quoting* S. Steib, *Engaging Families in Child Welfare Practice*, CHILDREN'S VOICE (2004), *available at* http://66.227.70.18/programs/r2p/cvarticlesef0409.htm)).

Finally, the role of denial of illness must be considered. In this case both AL, his mother and to some degree his father, engaged in denial, though with some vacillation (mother acknowledged concerns in various emails as did AL himself). The roots of denial run deep. Some originate in the individual and family system's psychological need, but certainly the stigma attaching to mental illness is a large contributor to the minimization of psychopathology.

The traditional model of service delivery for children with mental health, medical, developmental, or behavioral difficulties has been to ask "what is wrong with this child and what will we do about it, how will we treat him?" Little attention had historically been paid to the family itself, its needs, strengths and challenges, and how the system of the family contributes to or even unintentionally creates barriers to the wellness of the child.

> Increasingly we have come to understand that children's wellness does not exist in a vacuum, and that the caregivers' and children's well-being and healthy development are inextricably bound.[103]

We also increasingly appreciate that families need assistance in navigating the sometimes complex system of support that is available to help their children. This is why a mental health provider or even medical provider may provide care coordination to help a family identify and access appropriate services and to ensure continuity of information and support.

However, these family-centered approaches are still relatively new and certainly not routinely offered to children and their caregivers. Our medical and mental health care systems can still struggle to provide effective services to children in the context of the family, whether due to resource or reimbursement barriers.

Providers must have the staffing and financial supports to deliver family-focused support and care coordination. Providers must be reimbursed for and encouraged to provide appropriate support, care coordination, and referral for families. Services for children and families must be sustained, rather than episodic and periodic. The duration of services must be tied to measurable outcomes rather than predetermined fee for service schedules.

Many of these engagement strategies described herein could be offered by the educational system as well. Increasingly we must see our school systems as community providers for children *and* their families. We must also recognize that supporting children's social and emotional wellness is part of the job of schools as well as pediatricians, social workers, and mental health specialists.

To effectively engage and partner with parents, including those that may seem directive or difficult to reach, school systems, like community mental health or medical providers must have the resources, including space, personnel and expertise, to meaningful communicate with caregivers regarding the wellness of their children.

---

[103] *Id.* at 12–14 (discussing various examinations of the need to engage whole family system in therapeutic work with children.)

Additional Recommendations

<u>Education</u>

- Schools must play a critical role in the identification and referral of students with social, emotional, and behavioral health problems. This identification and referral is critical to ensure that students are then connected with the appropriate supports both in the school and in the home. Schools are "the *de facto* setting for connection to and provision of behavioral health services."[104] The goal of interconnection between separate systems within the mental health arena can only be successfully achieved through the integration of schools and their active participation concerning the mental health and wellness of their students.

- Increasingly, we recognize that school staff must have training to identify mental health warning signs: training can be provided through pre-certification curriculum, continuing education, and newer models such as Mental Health First Aide.

- While the identification of warning signs is important, teachers and school districts must also have the network and resources to refer and possibly coordinate services for the child and family.

- Schools must ensure that they are evaluating children in all areas of suspected disability, including conducting social-emotional evaluations. This is particularly critical for a student with known or suspected ASD, *even when* academic concerns are neither raised nor immediately evident.

- Schools must have capacity to address social-emotional learning, offer evidence-based social skills curriculum, skill building regarding social pragmatics, and therapeutic and behavioral supports by qualified professionals.

- Schools should have support and greater flexibility to import therapeutic and other related services (such as occupational therapy and behavior support services) into the school setting and mechanisms for Medicaid and private insurance reimbursement for delivered services should be established.

- The educational planning process must include participation of appropriate experts in all domains of development or disability. For a child such as AL, the team should consist of individuals who have expertise in working with children with neurodevelopmental disorders and co-occurring mental health disorders. A team of professionals may include a developmental specialist, clinical social worker, psychologist, behaviorist, and psychiatrist, as well as the special education teachers.

- State/s can provide more specific guidance to districts regarding what professionals must participate in the educational planning for children with emotional disturbance or autism, and how to identify and obtain relevant medical or mental health information for educational planning processes.

- Special education plans must include accurate information about a child's current levels of performance, goals, and clear objectives in all areas of need and anticipated growth. Success

---

[104] Sandra M. Chafouleas, *Effective School Discipline Policies and Practices (PPT)*, Congressional Briefing Presentation (2013).

rates and progress must be measured by more than observation, but garnered through a data-driven, quantitative and qualitative approach.

- Schools should ensure awareness of existing community resources and how to connect staff and families with available services. Notification alone is insufficient, however. Follow-up, ongoing care coordination and surveillance are also necessary. In AL's case, if this continuity of care were available it would have highlighted problems with treatment access or compliance much earlier in his developmental trajectory.

- Schools must have capacity to develop and provide comprehensive, individualized transition planning for youth with Autism Spectrum Disorders through age 21, with a focus on supporting a transition to independence where possible through development of independent living skills and connection with community supports.

- Districts should evaluate and annually report regarding the identified needs of special education students in their schools and indicate what resources, including personnel and research-based interventions, are being utilized within the district to support children in *all areas of disability.*

- While we cannot tell if AL experienced bullying, we do know that children with disabilities are particularly vulnerable to mistreatment at the hands of peers. The Department of Education and local school districts should be supported in their continuing efforts to combat bullying by the application of evidenced based school wide interventions and zero tolerance policies and regulations.

- School districts, alongside and with the support of the State Department of Education, should commit to a quality assurance and continued quality improvement program that focuses on compliance with educational best practices and state regulatory requirements. School districts can be supported with feedback and where appropriate, performance improvement plans.

- It is also vital to state that the lack of multi-disciplinary and individualized transition planning is a common and systemic concern, not unique to AL's IEP. Much more attention needs to be paid to post-secondary readiness for disabled youth and young adults, with a focus not only on academic skills but the ability to live as independently as possible, with or without community supports. The Connecticut State Department of Education published guidance, dated 2006-07, regarding appropriate transition planning for disabled students.[105]

The Role of Pediatrics

- Pediatricians' offices must have resources to conduct comprehensive and ongoing developmental and behavioral health screening for youth, with appropriate reimbursement strategies to support this work.

- Children and their families should have access to quality care coordination, often reserved only for children with complex medical needs, but beneficial for children with developmental challenges and mental health concerns. Care coordination should facilitate more effective information-sharing between medical, community, and educational providers.

---

[105] Connecticut State Department of Education, *Topic Brief: Writing Transition Goals and Objectives (2006-07)* http://www.sde.ct.gov/sde/cwp/view.asp?a=2626&q=322676 (Nov. 14, 2014).

- Pediatricians and related health professionals should be prepared to educate families about mental health issues, including suicide and other self-harm substance abuse and bullying when appropriate.
- Pediatricians should also be able to assess a child's behavioral health needs, provide primary mental health care with consultation as needed and make appropriate referrals to mental health specialists.

Supporting Children and Youth with Autism Spectrum Disorders and Co-Occurring Mental Health Disorders

A major issue faced by AL and his family was the paucity of services and supports for children and youth, particularly older youth and adults, who have Autism Spectrum Disorders with or without co-occurring mental health challenges. There is no indication, however, that the Lanzas sought ongoing mental health evaluation and treatment for AL in the last years of his life. Additionally, even if the IEP team had provided extended services for AL, the school district would also have had some difficulty connecting AL to community services that were appropriate for his needs post-graduation.

There are several challenges worth noting here. There is a dearth of evidence-based interventions for transition-age youth (a report for the Centers for Medicare and Medicaid Services in 2011 noted that only 7% of interventions identified for transition age youth met evidence-based standards, and that few interventions overall existed.)[106] [107] In fact, in a multi-state review conducted by the federal government, a lack of services (or access to services) for transition-age youth was identified by many states as the largest gap in services for individuals with autism spectrum disorders.[108]

Additionally, there remains a lack of professional expertise regarding autism spectrum disorders in the existing community-provider network, inclusive of pediatricians, mental health, and educational providers. For example, a report to the American Academy of Pediatrics in 2009 indicated that pediatricians felt less able to provide quality care to children with autism than to children with other complex conditions.[109] Primary care physicians also reported significant problems nationally in accessing specialists such as child and adolescent psychiatrists for consultation and assistance.[110]

Research confirms that many children with autism spectrum disorders may develop mental health disorders such as anxiety, attention deficit hyperactivity disorder, and depression, and that these

---

[106] D. MAUCH, ET AL., CENTERS FOR MEDICARE & MEDICAID SERVICES ASD SERVICES PROJECT, REPORT ON STATE SERVICES TO INDIVIDUALS WITH AUTISM SPECTRUM DISORDERS (April 1, 2011), *available at* http://www.google.com/url?sa=t&rct=j&q=&esrc=s&source=web&cd=5&ved=0CEAQFjAE&url=http%3A%2F%2Fwww.cms.gov%2Fapps%2Ffiles%2F9-state-report.pdf&ei=4ZohVO7CB5CTyASMi4Fo&usg=AFQjCNGlz8y46eLwk_sZQZpS7_ksSgw0HA&bvm=bv.75775273,d.aWw.

[107] This data compared to 31 interventions identified for young children, with about half meeting criteria for evidence-based service, and another 42% that were rated as "emerging evidence-based." *Id.* at 3.

[108] *Id.* at 7, 18, 32–33.

[109] *Id.* at 24 (*citing* Golnik et al., *Medical Homes for Children with Autism: A Physician Survey*, 123 PEDIATRICS 996, 966–71 (2009)).

[110] *Id.* at 24, n.29 (*citing* Cunningham, *Beyond Parity: Primary Care Physicians' Perspective on Access to Mental Health Care*, 28 HEALTH AFFAIRS 490, 490–501 (2009)).

children may be *more at risk* for developing mental health challenges than children who do not have these types of developmental differences.[111] Physicians and community health and mental health providers must be knowledgeable about the prevalence rate of ASD and associated mental health diagnoses so that children can be screened or evaluated for relevant conditions and increase their likelihood of appropriate diagnosis and treatment.

Schools and Children with Autism and Co-Occurring Mental Health Disorders

Schools may not be well equipped to identify, evaluate, and effectively serve children and youth with autism spectrum disorders, with or without co-occurring mental health disorders. With the relatively recent and dramatic increase in children who are diagnosed as having ASD, all community providers, including school districts, are coming to terms with their respective abilities and obligations to better identify and serve children with complex developmental and mental health profiles.

As stated throughout this report, schools have the obligation under state and federal laws to identify, evaluate, and provide evidence-based services to children with any type of disability that is impacting their ability to learn. However, authors acknowledge the dramatic workforce development needs, increased technical support, and expertise that will be required to help schools meaningfully meet their obligations and priorities with regard to children with complex developmental or mental health disorders.

Increase Access to Effective Interventions for Children and Youth with Autism

States must examine funding strategies to increase effective service delivery for children and transitioning youth with autism and related challenges.

Current strategies include state plans, Medicaid waivers, and increased insurance coverage for community-based supports. It is imperative to note, however, that not all children and their families are covered by insurance plans subject to the mandates of the Affordable Care Act, and that a percentage of children are covered by employer-sponsored plans that may be exempt from newer insurance mandates.[112]

Though many states, including Connecticut, now mandate insurance coverage for diagnosis and treatment of ASD, there remains a paucity of available services. Services must be created and targeted

---

[111] Center for Autism & Related Disabilities, University of South Florida, AUTISM & MENTAL HEALTH ISSUES: A GUIDEBOOK ON MENTAL HEALTH ISSUES AFFECTING INDIVIDUALS WITH AUTISM SPECTRUM DISORDER 4–6 (2009), available at http://card-usf.fmhi.usf.edu, at 4-6. *See also* S.E. Levy, et al., *Autism Spectrum Disorder and Co-Occurring Developmental, Psychiatric, and Medical Conditions Among Children in Multiple Populations of the United States*, 31 J. DEV. BEHAV. PEDIATR. 267, 267–75 (2010).

[112] Association of Maternal and Child Health Programs, ISSUE BRIEF: THE AFFORDABLE CARE ACT AND CHILDREN AND YOUTH WITH AUTISM SPECTRUM DISORDER AND OTHER DEVELOPMENTAL DISABILITIES 6 (2012) ("It is important to note that many of the reforms described above **do not apply** to two types of private health insurance plans: ***grandfathered plans and certain employer-sponsored plans,*** which are plans that were in effect on the day ACA was signed into law … are exempt from many of the health care reform law provisions as long as they keep their grandfathered status.") (emphasis added).

specifically for individuals with autism spectrum disorders who may need chronic, community-based supports.

The federal government's 2011 Medicare and Medicaid report on the status of autism spectrum services in multiple states acknowledged the "universal call" from states that the federal government support development of a public health response to individuals with autism in the following ways:

- Building a national ASD knowledge network or learning community to advance the capacity of state systems;
- Creating a national resource center to serve as a state information exchange;
- Issuing federal guidance on adoption and reimbursement of evidence-based/promising practices for ASD.[113]

In Connecticut, there have been several recent developments supporting improvement of access to services for individuals with Autism and their families. The Department of Developmental Services (DDS) is currently rolling out efforts to train and credential providers, increase services, and help families navigate the still fragmented system of care. Additionally, following a recent federal mandate to provide behavioral services to children and adolescents with autism, the Department of Social Services and DDS are establishing Medicaid support for this form of treatment.

Ensuring early diagnosis and comprehensive evaluation will also be imperative to improving treatment outcomes for children and youth with autism and related mental health disorders. In Connecticut, for example, the state's Birth to Three Program (IDEA Part C) delivers intensive in-home support specifically for children identified as having an Autism Spectrum Disorder, with screening for Autism taking place at 16 months of age.[114] These programs provide supports to the child and his or her caregivers multiple days per week, multiple times per day. Not every state is providing this level of early intervention for children with autism, which is the time of life when evidence confirms the highest level of efficacy for services is necessary.

2010 THROUGH 2012

After AL officially graduated from Newtown High School in 2009, he further retreated from virtually all structured community activities. He withdrew into a solitary physical and psychological existence, marked by hours in his room, extensive cyber-activities, and markedly decreased communication with family members. The record provides very little sense of his goals and objectives for his life during this time.

After AL began declining to spend time with Mr. Lanza, Mr. Lanza would regularly send emails to him asking him how he was doing. He asked AL to join him at events or other activities they had previously enjoyed, including arcades, shooting ranges, or coin shows. AL stopped sending any response to Mr. Lanza's emails sometime in 2010.

---

[113] D. MAUCH, *supra* note 97, at 7, n. 80.
[114] CONNECTICUT BIRTH TO THREE: SERVICE GUIDELINE FOR AUTISM SPECTRUM DISORDER: INTERVENTION GUIDANCE FOR SERVICE PROVIDERS (2011), http://www.birth23.org/.

The falling out between AL and Mr. Lanza may have been related to AL's desire to take college courses at Norwalk Community College. AL wanted to carry a full course load but Mr. Lanza said he couldn't handle that and wasn't being realistic. This may have been the last time that AL and Mr. Lanza actually spoke or emailed reciprocally. Mr. Lanza continued to let AL know that he wanted to see him:

> Sept. 18, 2010: "AL, I am very happy to hear from your mother that you are enjoying your classes. I hope that we can spend some time together soon, just let me know when you are available (even if only for a short period of time). Dec. 2, 2010:[115] "Hi. AL- I miss seeing you. I hope all is well with you. Let me know if and when you would like to shooting or go on a hike."

> June 16, 2011: "AL-Please respond to this email if you like to go on a hike. It would be interesting to see the status of the demolition work on the peninsula in Bridgeport."

> July 13, 2011: "Hi AL-Just a note to say "Hi", Please confirm receipt."

> Nov.18, 2011: (Mr. Lanza to Mrs. Lanza) ". . . I think you should tell [AL] that he should plan to see me once per month to do something (hike, cross country ski, shooting etc.)"

> Nov. 15, 2012 (From Mrs. Lanza to Mr. Lanza): "I will talk to him about that but I didn't want to harass him. He has had a bad summer and actually stopped going out. He wouldn't even go to the grocery store, so it's been pretty stressful. Yesterday was the first time in moths [sic] I've been able to talk him into going to do his own shopping and his car battery was actually dead because it sat so long. I ended up spending most of the day getting it fixed and now I am going to have to start pressuring him to go out all over again."

The last emails Mr. Lanza sent to AL were in the fall of 2012. Mr. Lanza specifically remembered asking AL to join him for a coin show in New Haven. AL never responded to his father's request. Mr. Lanza stated, in later police interviews, that although AL did not respond, Mr. Lanza would still make it a point to reach out to him at least six or eight times in the course of a year, offering different activities including skiing, shooting, or hiking. It does not appear that Mr. Lanza ever came to the house to confront or engage AL in any way about their lack of contact.

There is no indication that Mr. Lanza concluded that AL's mental or physical health had significantly deteriorated or that Mr. Lanza sought to facilitate a mental health intervention. In later interviews, Mr. Lanza indicated that he felt Mrs. Lanza was a contributing factor to AL distancing himself from him. Mr. Lanza stated that Mrs. Lanza often said that AL was doing well or better, and that the email in November that he was having great difficulty came as a surprise. Mr. Lanza noted that Mrs. Lanza did not tell other family members about the depths of what Mr. Lanza called AL's "seclusion." After

---

[115] Authors are providing excerpts or examples of emails sent by Mr. Lanza. These excerpts are not the complete universe of emails sent during this time period.

the shootings on December 12, 2012, Mr. Lanza spoke to a close relative of Mrs. Lanza's who also confirmed that Mrs. Lanza had not shared the gravity of AL's presentation in the waning months of his life.

People who knew Mrs. Lanza described her as spending a lot of time in a local restaurant and bar during this last year. According to one individual, Mrs. Lanza was often at the bar and she would stay late. When asked about AL and son Ryan, Mrs. Lanza would rarely speak about AL. Interviews indicate that Mrs. Lanza may have expressed some concern to friends or acquaintances about AL, particularly in 2012, noting that he had not come out of his room for months and that he would not engage with her. She worried that he did not care about her at all.

AL Became Increasingly Involved in Dance Dance Revolution

One activity that AL continued to engage in regularly during this time was "Dance Dance Revolution," a video game that he played at a local theater (and at home) and that he could play on his own or with others, where the user is required to move their feet rhythmically in response to video cues. Medical records as far back as 2003 document that he played this "exercise/dance game" for recreation.

For a time in his adolescence, AL engaged in this activity on his own or with his brother. Even through 2011, he was seen engaging in this activity with at least two other people. He played DDR so often that regulars at the theater where he played referred to him as the "DDR guy."

Reports were that AL would dance for hours at a time. Per description, he would whip himself into a frenzy, a behavior consistent, possibly, with a need to contain anxiety-producing impulses and thoughts. There were days when he would not do anything else but Dance Dance Revolution. He generally would do it alone except for his one friend at the time. AL would sometimes engage in this activity for ten hours at a time. He would move until he was drenched in sweat, not eating for extended periods. He would then retreat into the bathroom and wipe himself off, sometimes returning to the activity once again.

It is reasonable to speculate from this behavior that AL's mental health was deteriorating and that he was living with very serious inner turmoil at this time. Dance Dance Revolution served as a complete distraction and perhaps a containing device, as he danced to a state of physical exhaustion, only to return home to his self-imposed isolation.

One witness indicated in later interviews that at one point he even asked AL if he was okay after he had played the game for a very long time. AL replied that he didn't have any more money but that he just didn't want to go home. The witness stated that he offered him some money so he could play a little longer, which AL accepted. Later the witness heard that the manager of the theater had to eventually unplug the game to get AL to leave, as if AL could become so lost in the activity that he would not respond to communication. AL seemed to be dividing his life between various forms of escape in which he made minimal personal contact with other human beings, either dancing to the point of physical exhaustion while noticeably oblivious to other people in the theater, or physically shut off from the outer world in his room while immersed in a fantasy cyber-world.

AL was acquainted with another adolescent that he played DDR with on a regular basis. They would meet a few times per month to either play the video game or go to the movies. AL and his friend talked about multiple topics, including computers, chimp society, human nature, morality, prejudice, and sometimes about his family. AL told his friend that he had a strained relationship with his mother.

AL would sometimes talk with this friend about the topic of mental health or depression, though he never indicated that he was diagnosed with anything. He did tell his friend that mental health issues were not a reflection of the character of a person, but were symptoms of something else going on inside a person.

In later police interviews, the friend reported that AL was capable of emotion, of laughing, smiling, and making jokes, though he was not overly expressive.

According to the friend, AL enjoyed nature and talked about going hiking on a few occasions.

AL and the friend also talked about their interest in mass murderers or serial killers, but this was just considered to be a mutual morbid interest. Both he and his acquaintance liked horror movies. In June of 2012, he and his primary acquaintance had a falling out and stopped spending time together.

AL began researching mass shootings on the computer in 2011. His interest accelerated until he appeared to be obsessed with the details and narratives of these shooters. He and cyber-acquaintances would write about their mutual interest in various shooters and incidents.

AL Increasingly Spent Time Alone With his Computer

AL continued to spend time, as he did in earlier adolescence, playing online games such as World of Warcraft (WOW). He appeared to play this game with an associated avatar.

Gaming consoles found in AL's home showed a history of games such as "Dynasty Tactics, "Kingdom Hearts, and "The Two Towers." These games are designed for teenagers and for console use only. Another console showed a history of "Call of Duty 2: Big Red One," "Call of Duty: Finest Hour," "Dead or Alive 3," "Halo," "Lego Star Wars, "Mech Assault," "Mercenaries," and others. He also played "Combat Arms" on his computer, another multiplayer, first person shooter game.

AL's Cyber-Communication

AL's increasing descent into a world where he communicated most often, and at times perhaps singularly, with members of a cyber-community, is a significant development.

> Nov. 17, 2010 (AL to Cyber-Acquaintance): "It's amazing how fast time passes. It's hard to believe that it's already been this long. I'm sorry about my mood over the summer. I was more depressed than I had ever been before. When I apologized for it, you said that I wasn't behaving disrespectfully and that I never had been, but I don't think I've ever been as kind toward you as you deserve. I don't know how much it ever seemed like it, but I've always really appreciated your friendship. I've pretty much been a complete loner

throughout my life but I'm sure that even if I had more friends, you'd still be my favorite person I've met. I'd like it if we could do something together again sometime. . . . Please email back and we could figure out something amazing."

Over the last months of AL's life he was also closely connected to a small community of individuals that shared his dark and obsessive interest in mass murder.

> July 23, 2012 (From AL to Cyber-Acquaintance): "My interest in mass murdered [sic] has been perfunctory for such a long time. The enthusiasm I had back when Virginia Tech happened feels like it's been gone for a hundred billion years. I don't care about anything. I'm just done with it all."

Acquaintances wrote back and forth regarding various sources of information about shootings, including school shootings. His peer and community influences, present through much of his life, at least in some fashion, through school and family, had largely gone away. Replacing these influences was a narrow group of peers who exerted no positive, regulating force on AL. Unlike normalizing influences and positive community peer groups, his cyber group would have had little willingness or ability to stop his dangerous trajectory or to offer cautioning feedback to him about his impulses. The emails exchanged between AL and members of this macabre online community offer a rather breathtaking reflection of a negative micro-society within our midst.

It may be that AL fostered and nurtured his obsessive interest in mass murder because there was no parental oversight of his online and electronic activities. While AL was over age 18, he remained at home in an apparent state of "despondency," and malnutrition. Authors cannot know whether Mrs. Lanza ever tried (and failed) to enter AL's room or take an interest, however supervisory, in his activities. Given that AL's technological capabilities were superior to those of his mother, it may be that she would not have been able to trace his footsteps. However, authors must emphasize that supervision and at least awareness of an adolescent's online activities is very important, particularly so when the youth's mental and physical well-being is already in question.

Moreover, there is a growing discussion in the healthcare community of the phenomenon of internet or videogame addiction.[116] However, there is no agreement regarding diagnostic criteria, and the DSM-5 does not yet recognize internet or videogame addiction as an independent diagnosis.[117] Research does show however that similar to addicted users of substances, cocaine for instance, there are neurobiological changes that can be observed in the brains of heavy internet users.[118] Some researchers have found that heavy or addictive video game usage has a deleterious impact on social-emotional functioning, with others finding that youth with Autism Spectrum Disorders or Attention Deficit Hyperactivity Disorder were more likely to engage in addictive computer or game play than

---

[116] P. Weigle, *Internet and Video Game Addiction: Evidence & Controversy*, 4 J. ADOLES PSYCH 80, 83 (2014) (although there is no recognition of internet or gaming addiction in the DSM-V, "there has been a significant body of research on these subjects published since the DSM workgroup's determination was made").

[117] *Id.* Additionally, research indicates that *average* media time for youth may be upwards of 7.5 hours per day. P. Weigle & D. Reid, *Helping Parents Promote Healthy and Safe Computer Habits*, 4 J. OF ADOLES PSYCH 92, 92 (2014) (citing a 2010 Kaiser Family Foundation Survey). "The American Academy of Pediatrics' Policy Statement (Am. Acad. of Pediatrics 2013) recommends that parents create a family home use plan that limits youth to 1 or 2 hours of total screen time per day." *Id.*

[118] Weigle, *supra* note 107, at 85.

typically developing peers.[119] Video game and internet addiction appear to be "highly comorbid with several other psychiatric disorders" including anxiety, depression, and obsessive compulsive challenges.[120]

Emerging recommendations to assist youth (and parents) with the deleterious effects of internet addiction or over-use include individual treatment, family therapy to increase the family's "cohesiveness," psycho-education for parents about the impact of heavy internet or gaming use, the treatment of co-morbid conditions, and greater structure of the youth's and family's time.[121] Placement of computer or gaming equipment in common areas of the home and monitoring of youth's time and usage are also recommended strategies.

Essay Regarding Pedophilia

At some point, AL crafted an undated and lengthy essay, which he identified as a college admission application text, outlining a position that pedophilia should not be considered abhorrent or illegal. His essay, academic in tone, references varying cultural norms across the span of time to support a premise that our modern day attitudes about pedophilia are arbitrarily constructed. Authors are careful to note that there are no other writings that speak to a preoccupation he may or may not have had with pedophilia. There are no records and there is no evidence that he had pedophiliac tendencies. Authors note that there is evidence that he was in possession of video pornography, but that the contents of the pornography was not pedophiliac in nature. It is possible that the essay he drafted constituted an academic exercise that was not submitted for review by any educational professional. As with the "Big Book of Granny", it was obsessive in both length and tone, 34 pages long even though he stated that the "requirement" was 500 words.

Medical Records

AL transitioned to adult internal medicine by 2010. Records from his annual examination and a later visit in 2010 did not document any history of psychiatric issues or any significant presentation at the time of the visit. However, a note from December 2010 indicates that the primary care office received a call from Mrs. Lanza, who had apparently opened a letter addressed to AL from the healthcare provider notifying him of increased liver functions. Mrs. Lanza was noted to be "very upset," insisted on speaking with the doctor's office, and stated that AL would not talk on the phone so that an office visit would be required. AL then reported in the office visit the next day that he felt well generally. His weight was noted to be 120 pounds. AL's height was still 5 feet, 10 inches. The record documents that he was "alert," "well nourished," and "well developed." Additional lab studies were requested.

A February 2010 medical record notes nothing remarkable about AL's presentation. However, other indications regarding AL's presentation at this time, indicate that he was tall, very thin, and would not make eye contact.

---

[119] *Id.*
[120] *Id.* at 86.
[121] *Id.* at 89.

An email exchange between Mr. and Mrs. Lanza in 2011 indicates that further doctor visits may have occurred and may have addressed AL's fatigue. Available billing records indicate office visits through 2010, with lab work and a radiology visit in 2011.

Books

An inventory of books, likely belonging to or read and referenced by AL and found in his room by law enforcement investigators, included:

"American Military History and the Evolution of Western Warfare"
"Behind Hitler's Lines"
"Death and Taxes"
"Grimm Fairy Tales"
"No Surrender; My Thirty-Year War"
"Notes of a Revolutionary"
"OBA: The Last Samurai"
"Practical Shooting: Beyond Fundamentals"
"Ratman's Notebooks"
"Reflections of A Warrior"
"Salt: A World History"
"Strange Stories, Amazing Facts"
"The Anti-Federalist Papers and the Constitutional Convention Debates"
"The Glock in Competition"
"The Jungle is Neutral"
"The Sledge Patrol"
"The Sorrows of Young Werther"
"We Die Alone"

Anorexia

The Office of the Chief Medical Examiner found that at death, AL was anorexic (six feet tall and 112 pounds), to the point of malnutrition and resultant brain damage. This finding raises questions regarding how he, living at home and spending the majority of his time on his own, physically presented to his mother. Authors cannot determine what, if any, concerns were raised by his family regarding his eating ability or habits, or his continued emaciation during this time. AL's mother had consulted with his pediatrician years earlier about his weight, and by 2008, he was prescribed Miralax for ongoing constipation issues.

However, there is no indication that AL's family expressed concern to a mental health or medical professional between 2010 and 2012 regarding his malnutrition or any other issue. There are no medical records that indicate he was ever diagnosed with anorexia prior to his death or was being provided treatment of any kind for that condition. Anorexia, Obsessive Compulsive Disorder, and autism are conditions that individually increase the risk of suicide.[122] Anorexia can produce cognitive

---

[122] S. Mayes, et. al, *Suicide Ideation and Attempts in Children with Autism*, 7 RESEARCH IN AUTISM SPECTRUM DISORDERS 109, 109–19 (2013); N.L. Zucker, et al., *Anorexia Nervosa and Autism Spectrum Disorders: Guided Investigation*

impairment and it is likely that anorexia combined with an autism spectrum disorder and OCD compounded AL's risk for suicide.

Mrs. Lanza Planned to Move Away from Sandy Hook

Mrs. Lanza indicated an intention to move from Newtown to either Washington or North Carolina. She talked to AL about this move and apparently he indicated he would move to Washington with her. She planned to purchase an RV (Recreational Vehicle) so that she could show the house without AL living in it. AL would live in the RV instead while the house was on the market. Mrs. Lanza told a friend that if she moved to Washington State, she would try to enroll him in a "special school." She also stated that she wanted him to learn to be more self-sufficient.

AL Became Increasingly Isolated

A friend of Mrs. Lanza's talked about how AL seemed to become, according to his mother, increasingly despondent. He had not left his room for approximately three months and Mrs. Lanza indicated that she was addressing his every need, though she and her son communicated only via e-mail. Mrs. Lanza appeared to attribute all of his presentation to his Asperger's Syndrome, and she felt that he had no emotional connection to her.

Despite AL's not having left the home for months, and despite Mrs. Lanza's growing and stated concern for his wellbeing, it does not appear that Mrs. Lanza communicated these concerns to any mental health or medical professional.

Final Months before Tragedy

After an exhaustive review of records, emails, and conclusions drawn by law enforcement agencies, authors conclude that AL was not obviously psychotic in the time period leading up to the Sandy Hook shooting, though he had a history of depression and suicidal ideation that can be seen in his emails during 2011 and 2012.

The FBI Behavior Analysis Unit determined after an exhaustive forensic review of AL's computer usage that his obsession and attention to detail with mass killing was *unprecedented.*

By the summer of 2012 he had stopped seeing his one and only friend after a dispute over a movie.

AL sustained and injury to his head the night before Mrs. Lanza left for a trip to New Hampshire— 2 or 3 days prior to the Sandy Hook shooting. Mrs. Lanza describes his injury in a text message reading "bloody, bloody, bloody." Mrs. Lanza went on her trip anyway, and returned on December 13, 2012.

The looming prospect of moving from Newtown may have increased AL's anxiety, as he may have worried about where he would go or live, and the loss of the sanctuary he had developed in his home. This was quite possibly an important factor leading to the shootings.

---

of Social Cognitive Endophenotypes, PSYCHOL. BULL. 976–1006 (Nov. 2007). Roberts, A.R., Yaeger, K., Seigel, A. *Obsessive-compulsive disorder, comorbid depression, substance abuse, and suicide attempts: clinical presentations, assessments, and treatment. Brief Treatment and Crisis Intervention* 3:2. Summer 2003.

Authors conclude that there was not one thing that was necessarily the tipping point driving AL to commit the Sandy Hook shooting. Rather there was a cascade of events, many self-imposed, that included: loss of school; absence of work; disruption of the relationship with his one friend; virtually no personal contact with family; virtually total and increasing isolation; fear of losing his home and of a change in his relationship with Mrs. Lanza, his only caretaker and connection; worsening OCD; depression and anxiety; profound and possibly worsening anorexia; and an increasing obsession with mass murder occurring in the total absence of any engagement with the outside world. AL increasingly lived in an alternate universe in which ruminations about mass shootings were his central preoccupation.

The attack on Sandy Hook Elementary appears to have been a **purposefully thought-out and planned attack—AL did not just "snap."** He visited the school's website on numerous occasions. He had looked at the student handbook and viewed security procedures at the school.

According to the FBI, shooters are likely to target places or people that are familiar to them. AL would walk to Sandy Hook Elementary School with his father long after he stopped going to school there. The elementary school may have been targeted because he could overpower people, a dynamic that is very important for mass shooters as they do not want to be thwarted.

AL appears to have been on a path to violence for some time. The more rigid he became, the harder he was to reach. His world began to shrink at an accelerating rate, filled in only with details of horrifying events. Over the years when he became distressed, he became hypervigilant, keenly aware of and prone to perseverate about potential threats. He also became emotionally dysregulated and would cope by withdrawing into a detached private inner world either physically (spending days on end in his dark room and dancing manically) or psychologically. When distressed, he also became immersed in hostility-dominated fantasies that blurred the boundaries between inner experience and outer reality.

Authors infer that AL felt increasing anxiety, perhaps desperate about the potential loss of his sanctuary—the family home—and his caregiver moving on with her life. Reviewing whatever can be known about him at this time in his life, one can readily conclude that he felt totally incapable of adapting to a new environment, no less living on his own.

If Mrs. Lanza was going to withdraw his "prosthetic environment" (using Yale Child Study Center's much earlier observation), then AL might well have felt that he had no option left but to escape into death. It may be these fears, combined with his pervasive ruminations about mass shootings, (and the acceptance and encouragement of these by an online group of like-minded peers) that pushed him from fantasy into action.

Authors believe it was important to know as much as possible about AL's mental state during the last period of his life so as to better inform clinical conclusions and recommendations. Our capacity to know with any certainty, however, is severely limited by the paucity of information. We do know that, by this point, AL was living alone in his room with black plastic garbage bags on the windows, a locked door, and was communicating little with the outside world.

Though this picture could suggest a possible psychotic break, a review of emails authored by AL through the last days of his life suggests that his thinking, while highly idiosyncratic and verging on the bizarre with regard to mass murder, was not actively psychotic.[123]

There is evidence that AL lived a significant portion of this time in the cyber world, and that within that world he communicated his obsession with mass shootings as in the following email written three days before the Sandy Hook tragedy.

It is possible that he increasingly lost touch with reality as a result of this profound isolation and immersion in violence-filled fantasy worlds that he shared with others.

From: (AL)
Date: 12/11/2012 9:56pm
To: xxxxxxxxxxxxxx

I didn't really look at the emails you sent earlier, so I guess I ought to respond now. About the Chinese mass stabbers, they blend together in my mind too much for me to say much. Although I guess that should make it even easier to talk about them…I don't know. Who am I to even say anything on the topic? The inexplicable mystery to me isn't how there are massacres, but rather how there aren't 100,000 of them every year. So when it comes to rates and such, causes and consequences, domestic or forging (sic), in whatever context, I'm just going to be completely making things up because I apparently don't understand any of it.

I'm clueless about Olga Hepnarova. While granting that modus operandi really isn't that important, I just can't get into vehicular slaughterers. It seem too mediated, like using remote explosives (too hot). And knives stray too far from the whole "mass" aspect (too cold). The aesthetic of pistols tends to be just (sic) right.

A list of mass shooter suicide notes…I never thought to compile such a thing before. I can't remember ever thinking, "Whoa, that guy had a suicide note and I'm just finding out about this?! If their existence is every (sic) divulged by the police, it tends to be pretty public knowledge; and if their contents are released, they're even more prominent. So I'm probably not privy to any information that you aren't' already well-aware of. All I can offer is to say that you can probably rest easy knowing that you aren't overlooking too many lurking Jiverlys.

As far as the Holmies go…well, the .gif of him dancing on a llama was cute. I guess that's all I can say about the whole Holmie thing since I can't really relate to it. I don't understand why there weren't the "he's just a poor misunderstood puppy who needs help" type flocking around Jared Loughner since that spiel ostensibly applied to him more than James Holmes. And speaking more generally, I don't really understand why Aurora shooting was considered such a big deal all-around, as if such a thing had never happened before. It's not like its 1984.

---

[123] A review of the emails that AL sent to others during these last months and weeks were determined to be very useful in assessing whether AL was indeed psychotic at this time in his life. These emails were ultimately made available to the Office of the Child Advocate and referenced by authors for the purpose of creating this report.

FINAL STATEMENT

AL's deterioration ultimately led to his horrendous actions on December 14, 2012 when he carried out a planned attack on Sandy Hook Elementary School, murdering twenty-six innocent adults and children. Nothing can mitigate or fully explain those actions. This report cannot offer solace or answers for the indescribable pain and trauma inflicted by AL.

This report raises, but cannot definitively answer, the question as to whether better access to effective mental health and educational services would have prevented the tragic events at Sandy Hook. It is important to emphasize that AL's developmental condition and mental health cannot be seen as determinative of his extreme violent behavior.

The records herein reviewed support the presence of early developmental challenges consistent with a form of autism. There is also considerable evidence pointing to mental health issues beyond autism, such as an anxiety disorder, Obsessive Compulsive Disorder, and suicidal ideation. Children with this type of constitutional vulnerability combined with complex family dynamics as well as dual diagnosis present many treatment challenges. Going further, and most importantly, there is also evidence of primitive anger and preoccupation with violence. This aspect presents the strongest connection to AL's actions. Authors cannot know the source of such preoccupation **and there is no connection in the literature between AL's developmental profile and an increased likelihood of violent actions**.

The likelihood of an individual with Autism Spectrum Disorder and/or severe problems with anxiety and obsessive compulsive tendencies committing an act of pre-meditated violence, much less one of AL's magnitude, is rare. Individuals with these mental health or developmental disorders are more likely to internalize (that is, to feel distressed emotionally or to be confused, socially inappropriate or inept, and sometimes to harm themselves inadvertently or intentionally) than to externalize (that is, to act out aggressively so as to harm others).

In AL's case, his severe and deteriorating internalized mental health problems were combined with an atypical preoccupation with violence that had been evident at least since he authored the Big Book of Granny, and that appeared to be exacerbated by access to a segment of the cyber-world in which mass violence was a dominant theme of intellectualized speculation and debate, and horribly, fascination and celebration. Combined with access to deadly weapons, this proved a recipe for mass murder. Autism Spectrum Disorder or other psychiatric problems neither caused nor led to his murderous acts.

Authors cannot definitively answer questions regarding "why" AL committed mass murder, or whether, if more had been provided to him or for him, his terrible actions could have been prevented. However, after careful review of AL's records, authors observe that gaps or insufficiencies in professional-family communication and services can lead to severe deterioration in children and young adults with serious emotional disturbance. Such deterioration, while *rarely leading to such catastrophic events as in Sandy Hook*, may still produce outcomes that nevertheless are extremely harmful and costly to the youth, his or her family, and to the community and society.

It is fair to surmise that, had AL's mental illness been adequately treated in the last years of his life, one predisposing factor to the tragedy of Sandy Hook might have been mitigated. Although parents and other legal guardians ultimately are responsible for their children's health and safety, it is the educational and professional systems that must provide a safety net in instances where parents cannot or do not care successfully for a child.

This report in no way blames parents, educators or mental health professionals for AL's heinous acts, nor for his severe mental deterioration and extreme detachment from relationships with human beings, but authors point to the need for renewed vigilance by the child-serving professionals and systems to identify and ensure sufficient, effective services for the potentially tens of thousands of other children who slip between the cracks every year as a result of these types of problems.

AL's story highlights the need to address the profound gaps in our continuum of services for children with developmental and mental health needs, and further develop our capacity to provide carefully individualized, timely, and sustained assistance not only to children and young adults but also to their families, instead of waiting until severe crises or developmental failures (school drop-out, unemployment, divorce, homelessness, or delinquency) necessitate costly emergency services, the break-up of families, or the removal of children or adults from their families or society—as well as rarer mass tragedies.

It is also imperative that states and communities develop practices and policies that facilitate ready exchange of information from one system to another. All service agencies that intersect with children: schools, pediatricians, and mental health providers have responsibilities to support children's health and well-being, and we cannot continue to compartmentalize children's "mental health" into a singular program or service that may always be someone else's or some other entity's responsibility.

Holding systems accountable will require attention to appropriate resource allocation and utilization, including strengthening community mental health resources and the ability to flexibly import those services into home, schools, and other natural settings. But accountability will also require that we ably assess *the quality* of our service delivery, be it pediatric medical care, mental health evaluation, treatment, and special education services.

While authors' focus has been on AL's psychological deterioration, we reiterate that this should not be taken to mean that we do not recognize the ubiquitous role that guns, and especially assault weapons with high capacity magazines, play in mass murder. In fact, while mental illness plays only a small role in violence in America, assault weapons are an increasingly common denominator in violent crimes. The widespread access to assault weapons and high capacity ammunition is an urgent public health concern.

Finally, none of the findings in this report should be interpreted as exculpating or reducing AL's accountability for his actions. Roughly twenty percent of adolescents and young adults suffer from a variety of mental illnesses.[124] Many of these are complex (with multiple diagnoses), treatment

---

[124] DR. ANDREA SPENCER, CENTER FOR CHILDREN'S ADVOCACY, BLIND SPOT: UNIDENTIFIED RISKS TO CHILDREN'S MENTAL HEALTH (2012), *available at* https://www.cthealth.org/wp-content/uploads/2011/04/2BlindSpot2012.pdf.

resistant, and accompanied by a multiplicity of severe and confounding psychosocial problems. And yet, only an infinitesimally small number of such individuals go on to commit murder.

While we describe the predisposing factors and compounding stresses in AL's life, **we do not conclude that they add up to an inevitable arc leading to mass murder.**

There is no way to adequately explain why AL was obsessed with mass shootings and how or why he came to act on this obsession. In the end, only he, and he alone, bears responsibility for this monstrous act.

APPENDIX
RELEVANT LAWS REGARDING MENTAL HEALTH AND EDUCATIONAL SERVICE DELIVERY

SPECIAL EDUCATION FOR CHILDREN, INCLUDING EARLY INTERVENTION

Federal law, namely the Individuals with Disabilities Education Act (IDEA), 20 U.S.C. § 1400 (2004), requires states to meet the developmental and educational needs of children, age birth to twenty, who have disabilities.

Under IDEA states are required to operate an effective early intervention service delivery model for infants and toddlers with disabilities, developmental delays, or medical conditions likely to lead to developmental challenges (IDEA Part C). IDEA also requires that early intervention programs identify and provide services for children who have developmental delays in the area of *social-emotional* development as well.

Once a child reaches three years of age, federal law requires that school districts identify and evaluate children with suspected disabilities, even without an affirmative request from the child's parent or guardian (though parental consent is required).

Identification of a Child with a Disability

Special education law identifies various areas of eligibility for special education services, and these areas include (but are not necessarily limited to): autism spectrum disorders, communication disorders, deaf-blindness, developmental delay, emotional disabilities, hearing impairments, learning disabilities, multiple disabilities, orthopedic impairment, other health impairment, traumatic brain injury, and others.

Multidisciplinary Evaluation

A child suspected of having a disability that is interfering with their ability to learn should receive a *multidisciplinary* evaluation so that the child can be assessed in all areas of suspected disability and have an educational program that is tailored to meet their needs in multiple domains of development. For example, a child presenting with a speech delay may also require a social-emotional evaluation to see how the communication delay may be affecting the child's development in other domains.

Determination of Special Education Eligibility

The decision as to whether a child is eligible for special education and related services is based both on evaluations and the opinions and assessments of all members of the child's Individualized Education Plan team. This team includes the parent, the school administrators, district representatives, relevant evaluators, and teachers. A parent may bring their own ideas, evaluations, and priorities to the team meeting. These must be considered as part of the decision-making process. Indeed, all decisions made by the IEP team must include parental participation and input.

The Individual Education Plan

Once a child is identified as eligible (i.e. needing) for special education services, the IEP team (inclusive of the parent or guardian) comes together to create an Individualized Education Plan for the student. The IEP will document the nature of the child's disability, what related challenges the child has, what services and accommodations will be provided to the child to help them make progress in school, what goals and objectives the child is expected to achieve, and how the child's progress and achievement will be observed and evaluated. The IEP will also include a description of the child's current level of performance (in multiple domains, including academic and social-emotional) in various areas.

The IEP should specifically state what evidence-based services will be provided to the child, as well as the duration and frequency of such services. It is imperative that services are research-based and tailored to the child's *individual* needs. Federal law emphasizes individualization of services and education plans.

A child's IEP must also address whether the child needs school year round, called Extended Year Services. After a child turns 14, the IEP must include a statement of transition services, meaning how the child will be assisted in developing and preparing for life after high school. Transition services should be individualized to the strengths and interests of the child and include multidisciplinary supports, academic and experiential learning to help the child attain adequate academic, and functional living skills. These services can include everything from job coaching, shadowing, mentoring, to volunteering and life skills development.

The IEP must ensure that the child receives education in the least-restrictive environment appropriate to that child's needs. This means that a child may receive services in the mainstream class environment, modified with individual supports or accommodations. Sometimes, the "least restrictive environment" that is capable of meeting the child's needs for appropriate supports is a small, structured program with intensive services, run by either the school district or a private program paid for by the school district.

An IEP should address physical, cognitive, and social-emotional challenges displayed by the student.

The law also provides that parent training must be offered by the school district if this type of parent education is necessary for the child to make appropriate and expected progress in school.

Central themes underlying special education law are that the IEP must be the product of parental participation and team decision-making. The IEP must also be individualized to the needs of the child. There is no one-size fits all approach in special education.

Special Education Laws, Autism, Emotional Disturbance, and Other Health Impairment

As stated above, the law itself outlines what may be considered a disability qualifying a child for special education and related services.

"Autism" is defined in federal law as:

> A developmental disability significantly affecting verbal and nonverbal communication and social interaction, generally evident before age three, that adversely affects a child's educational performance. Other characteristics often associated with autism are engagement in repetitive activities and stereotyped movements, resistance to environmental change or change in daily routines, and unusual responses to sensory experiences.
>
> > (ii) Autism does not apply if a child's educational performance is adversely affected primarily because the child has an emotional disturbance, as defined in paragraph (c)(4) of this section.
> >
> > (iii)_A child who manifests the characteristics of autism after age three could be identified as having autism if the criteria in paragraph (c)(1)(i) of this section are satisfied. [125]

Emotional Disturbance is another category of disability giving rise to a child's eligibility for special education services.

"Emotional Disturbance" is defined as:

> A condition exhibiting one or more of the following characteristics over a long period of time and to a marked degree that adversely affects a child's educational performance:
>
> > (A) An inability to learn that cannot be explained by intellectual, sensory, or health factors.
> >
> > (B) *An inability to build or maintain satisfactory interpersonal relationships with peers and teachers.*
> >
> > (C) *Inappropriate types of behavior or feelings under normal circumstances.*
> >
> > (D) *A general pervasive mood of unhappiness or depression.*
> >
> > (E) A tendency to develop physical symptoms or fears associated with personal or school problems. [126]

---

[125] 34 C.F.R § 300.8(c)(1) (2013).
[126] 34 C.F.R § 300.7(c)(4) (2013) (emphasis added).

"Other health impairment" is defined as:

> Having limited strength, vitality, or alertness, including a heightened alertness to environmental stimuli, that results in limited alertness with respect to the educational environment, that--
>
> (i) Is due to chronic or acute health problems such as asthma, attention deficit disorder or attention deficit hyperactivity disorder, diabetes, epilepsy, a heart condition, hemophilia, lead poisoning, leukemia, nephritis, rheumatic fever, sickle cell anemia, and Tourette syndrome; and
>
> (ii) Adversely affects a child's educational performance.[127]

FEDERAL AND STATE PRIVACY LAWS: CONFIDENTIALITY OF INDIVIDUAL HEALTH RECORDS

Federal law outlines the privacy and confidentiality afforded to medical and mental health records. The federal Health Insurance and Portability and Accountability Act of 1996 (HIPAA) Pub.L. 104-191) provides that an individual's health information is confidential and can be shared without the consent of the individual (or the guardian) only under narrowly and strictly defined conditions and circumstances.

Federal confidentiality laws covers all types of medical providers, defined to include virtually all health organizations and service providers. Unless the subject of the record, or in the case of a minor, the guardian, consents to release of the information, the law rarely permits confidential information to be shared. Confidential information may be shared without necessary consent in the following relevant circumstances:

1. When the release of specific medical information is necessary for treatment purposes.
2. When an individual presents as an imminent threat to other people.
3. As otherwise required by state law, such as reporting of child abuse or neglect by health care providers or others.

CONFIDENTIALITY OF EDUCATIONAL RECORDS

The Federal Family Educational Rights and Privacy Act of 1974 (FERPA) 20 U.S.C. § 1232g, governs the confidentiality and sharing of educational records. All elementary and public schools, and most post-secondary colleges and universities, are subject to the provisions of FERPA. The default principle of FERPA is that educational records are private and confidential and cannot be shared without the consent of a parent (or adult student) unless otherwise permitted by law. It is important to note that FERPA covers the educational record itself and *not the observations or recollections of educational service providers.* A teacher concerned about the behavior of a particular student is not

---

[127] 34 C.F.R § 300.7(c)(9) (2013).

necessarily prohibited from informing others about the student's behavior. The observational concern itself is not covered by FERPA.

CONNECTICUT SCHOOL LAW: DUTIES OF PARENTS

Sec. 10-184. Duties of parents. School attendance age requirements. All parents and those who have the care of children shall bring them up in some lawful and honest employment and instruct them or cause them to be instructed in reading, writing, spelling, English grammar, geography, arithmetic and United States history and in citizenship, including a study of the town, state and federal governments. Subject to the provisions of this section and section 10-15c, each parent or other person having control of a child five years of age and over and under eighteen years of age shall cause such child to attend a public school regularly during the hours and terms the public school in the district in which such child resides is in session, unless such child is a high school graduate or the parent or person having control of such child is able to show that the child is elsewhere receiving equivalent instruction in the studies taught in the public schools. For the school year commencing July 1, 2011, and each school year thereafter, the parent or person having control of a child seventeen years of age may consent, as provided in this section, to such child's withdrawal from school. Such parent or person shall personally appear at the school district office and sign a withdrawal form. Such withdrawal form shall include an attestation from a guidance counselor or school administrator of the school that such school district has provided such parent or person with information on the educational options available in the school system and in the community. The parent or person having control of a child five years of age shall have the option of not sending the child to school until the child is six years of age and the parent or person having control of a child six years of age shall have the option of not sending the child to school until the child is seven years of age. The parent or person shall exercise such option by personally appearing at the school district office and signing an option form. The school district shall provide the parent or person with information on the educational opportunities available in the school system.

Sec. 10-184a. Special education programs or services for children educated in a home or private school. (a) The provisions of sections 10-76a to 10-76h, inclusive, shall not be construed to require any local, regional or state board of education to provide special education programs or services for any child whose parent or guardian has chosen to educate such child in a home or private school in accordance with the provisions of section 10-184 and who refuses to consent to such programs or services.

(b) If any such board of education provides special education programs or services for any child whose parent or guardian has chosen to educate such child in a private school in accordance with the provisions of section 10-184, such programs or services shall be in compliance with the Individuals with Disabilities Education Act, 20 USC 1400 et seq., as amended from time to time.

Regulations of Connecticut State Agencies (regarding homebound instruction, operative through 2013) Sec. 10-76d-15. Homebound and hospitalized instruction: A board of education shall provide homebound and hospitalized instruction when recommended by the planning and placement team.

(a) Requirements of individualized education program. Homebound and hospitalized instruction shall be as specified in the child's individualized education program, subject to the following.

> (1) In the case of a child not otherwise in need of special education and related services, homebound or hospitalized instruction shall maintain the continuity of the child's regular program. The requirements of evaluation and an individualized education program shall not apply and a planning and placement team meeting need not be convened.

> (2) In the case of a child not previously receiving special education and related services, the requirements of evaluation and an individualized education program shall apply if there is reason for the planning and placement team to believe that the child will continue to require special education and related services.

> (3) In the case of a child receiving special education and related services, the planning and placement team shall, where necessary, modify short-term instructional objectives in the child's individualized education program

(b) Necessary conditions. Homebound and hospitalized instruction shall be provided only when the planning and placement team finds that one or more of the following conditions applies.

> (1) A physician has certified in writing that the child is unable to attend school for medical reasons and has stated the expected date the child will be able to return to the school.

> (2) The child has a handicap so severe that it prevents the child from learning in a school setting, or the child's presence in school endangers the health, safety or welfare of the child or others.

> (3) A special education program recommendation is pending and the child was at home at the time of referral.

> (4) The child is pregnant or has given birth and a physician has certified that homebound or hospitalized instruction is in the child's best interest and should continue for a specified period of time.

(c) Length of absence. Homebound or hospitalized instruction shall be provided when a child's condition will cause an absence of at least three weeks' duration.

> Provided nothing in the child's condition precludes it, such instruction shall begin no later than two weeks from the first day of absence.

(d) Time and place. Homebound and hospitalized instruction shall be provided for at least one hour per day or five hours per week for children in grades kindergarten through six and at least two hours per day or ten hours per week for children in grades seven through twelve. Where evaluative data indicates that these time requirements are too great for the child, the planning and placement team may decrease instruction time. Instruction shall be provided in the setting of the child's home or the hospital to which the child is confined.

Printed in Great Britain
by Amazon

41388697R00068